First Published in Great Britain in 2020

ISBN 978-1-8380546-6-3
A Motiv8.me publication

Motiv8.me Press
Wrexham Enterprise Hub
11-13 Rhosddu Road
Wrexham
LL11 1AT

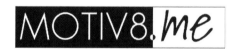

www.motiv8.me

# Self-Care for Givers and the Helping Professions

## Emma Sims

# Chapters

## Part 1

## Part 2

Acknowledgements

Bibliography

Reference Index

# About the Author

Emma Sims is a complementary Holistic Therapist and Reiki Master Teacher with 20+ years of experience in the field. She is based in the Community Resource Centre, Gwersyllt, Wrexham, North Wales.

She is the co-creator of Diamond Energy Therapy, Angelic Energy Therapy and her signature treatments include Heaven & Earth, Twinkle Toes, & Body Talk.

'Self-Care for Givers and the Helping Professions' is Emma's first book. It draws on her own lifelong experiences along with over fifteen years of experience as a therapist to help survivors, therapists and givers recognise the need to care for themselves, and offers a range of tried and tested techniques to help restore energy, balance and wellness.

# Dedication

To Poppy, Sue Winter & Dawn Knox for turning my life around so I could begin to self-care

# Foreword

For survivors, therapists and givers, who need a hefty compassionate kick up the rear!

In this book we look at not only methods or ways to promote our own self-care but the obstacles that might be stopping us from doing that. If burnout, weariness, irritability and over-giving is a facet in your life this book may be for you.

This is a book that you may well dip into, then put into practice, then fall down, then need more help and inspiration again so come back to. The journey is not linear and we may go back and forth between doing and not, as we learn to integrate. It is divided into two parts. The first section looks at obstacles that may be limiting your self-care and why you may stop yourself from doing what you 'know' you should be doing, but don't. Part two is a section you may wish to jump into for ideas, inspiration and a little bit of background information on ways to self-care.

Its timely that the release of the book coincides with the highlighted need for self-care during the pandemic. When we were advised that the NHS wouldn't be able to cope, many of us may have thought more about self-care, but not always known how to. The situation reminded me of the process of parentification, where the parents can't cope so the children take on more responsibility and an adult role which can ultimately create mental instability. There is also the concern that the impact of the self isolation has had on many and the feeling of institutionalisation and resulting anxiety that coming out of lockdown may have had. For some it has been a blessing which has highlighted a need to change, but how?

This overall call to grow can be beneficial in the longterm. Sales of immune support vitamins, according to a health food chain, have apparently increased during this time, which is a positive self care indicator. There is more need for us to take responsibility for our own health and do what we can to be well. Self-care might mean that we need to take action to call a GP during this current crisis to get checked out. It's been reported how less people picking up the phone could be the reason for a current decline in cancer diagnosis at the time of the pandemic. Please do get checked out if you need to!

I feel that there is much symbolism at this time, how events conspired to give people time out and brought many back to nature as part of their daily exercise. I thought about how Covid causes the problems with breathing, the lungs often associated holistically with grief. And how many of us do need to slow down and take a breath. And then came the masks. In spiritual and psychological development the mask is often referred to as the barrier to our true self, what we hide behind and what we cover up about ourselves, the face we put on for the world. Our words 'I'm fine' when really we aren't, mask how we really feel. So I invite you to take your metaphorical mask off and be true to yourself and whilst reading this book, take a breath, take time. As I have to remind myself to do too!

## Reflections on a self-care journey

I am a Holistic Therapist from North Wales, who through my own ongoing journey of healing has had to look at ways to self-care to help my own health. Now a self-confessed Queen of Self-Care, I know that even a good Queen falls off her throne at times. This can be a life long process and there's still much for me to learn too! I hope that insights gleaned from my journey and contained within this book help you in your own journey to receiving. Allowing yourself to do that and giving to yourself something is really rather obvious, but so many of us don't. In ten or twenty years time it will probably be old news, much more acceptable and we will all be 'Getting Melfish'. But here we are on the forefront of it.

## Getting Melfish?

The original title of this book was Getting Melfish. Reflecting back upon my diagnosis of M.E., I played with the symbolism of that. 'It's all about me', 'it needs to be about me', 'what about me?' etc., etc.; it really was directing me back to M.E., trying to understand who I was. I think, so I could understand how to take better care of myself. My intuition offered me the word 'Melfish'. I googled the meaning of the word 'fish'. It is defined as 'connecting us with the water element, it represents the deeper awareness of the unconscious or higher self', so the word Melfish itself would suggest that by paying attention to ourselves, to 'me' we can attain a deeper awareness of ourselves. So where does that leave the 'l', I literally heard the word 'learn' so l is for learn, Melfish ultimately means: 'I learn about ME to attain awareness of my unconscious or higher self'.

Melfish is the art of taking care of 'ME' and challenging the concept that it is selfish to take good care of ourselves. Recognising our needs, putting ourselves as a priority when previously we may not have. Understanding that if we do take care of us, we can take better care of others, particularly to prevent burnout. We cannot serve from an empty cup, but how often do we try?!

Melfish activities might include sitting down and having a quiet cup of tea, putting our feet up to recharge during the day when we might not normally do so, making sure we eat lunch sitting down, having a massage or therapy regularly, meditating, enjoying a lovely bubble bath with the door locked, taking a restorative walk in nature and many more which we will explore in this book. But most of us have barriers to this, we often have good intentions that we will begin to take better care of ourselves, that we will try to walk our talk, then fall at the first hurdle.

## It's all about M.E.

A little background as to how I came to write this book on self-care. Coming through my own journey of healing, which taught me the need for self-care and the obstacles encountered, as well as some of the struggles and observations I had and continue to have with that. I always say we teach what we need to learn and it is a journey!

## Self-Care for mind, body and spirit

So it was with a full heart that I started writing this book because that isn't always the case, nor has it always been that way. I'm still trying to walk that talk too. However, coming from a place of chronic illness and as a now therapist, I have literally learned the hard way and am still learning. We teach what we need to learn! Along the way I have accumulated a number of tools which have helped and I offer them in this book with gratitude for some of the things that I now know.

The suggestion that was given to me at the start of my more conscious journey was 'take what you need and dismiss the rest'. Whatever makes sense for you, go with, try it out experiment, experience, if not try something else. We are all different and all respond to things differently, that's part of our uniqueness.

For many of us self-care is something that we may have to learn, assigning ourselves the space to heal or replenish, whilst maybe battling with a part of ourselves that doesn't think that we are deserving or thinking that we are further down the list of priorities than everyone else. It is something that we may have to learn to do, to serve from a full heart filled cup rather than that empty one.

Self-care (SC) may not always come in the packages that we expect such as sitting down and having a massage or a bubble bath. It can spring forth in a myriad of smaller ways, which can be part of the jigsaw picture puzzle that is a whole new stronger you, once you put the pieces together. If you are tired and drained from life's challenges, chip away at this or dip into the book the best you can. This is often when we may most benefit. Handing the outcomes over to the powers that be, whoever you perceive them to be and asking for help if we are stuck and can't find a way through.

I wish you wellness and the cup that you will know how to replenish for yourself with the elixir of life force, on your journey forward, from now on.

## Beginnings

Suffice to say, like may of us on this path, I had a difficult ,unhappy childhood. On the surface I put on the brave face that many of us do, 'because that is what is expected of us'. I began to experience thoughts of self-harm around the age of eight. It didn't occur to me to tell anyone as that wasn't the done thing. I also had some amazing moments of insight, looking up at the stars and feeling ever so humble, and deep ponderings where I'd wonder how many people would fit into heaven and why it wasn't overcrowded and how does that work.

During my teens and onwards I was prescribed various antidepressants by well meaning physicians, but was continually struggling with depression and anxiety, as well as an inability to articulate myself, my emotions or my experiences. I didn't know who I was, or what I wanted. Therein started years of counselling with adolescent services and exploration to try to heal the black hole within.

## Hard Work

After leaving a degree course in Leeds, with depression and anxiety, I started my first job hoping that was the right course of action for me. However, after a while, I became even more unhappy and developed irritable bowel syndrome. One of my colleagues was picky and humiliated me on a number of occasions which, according to another colleague, was bullying. I didn't understand and had trouble accepting this because it had come to seem normal for me to be around people like that, and something I had experienced throughout my life. If we have always grown up around certain behaviour and don't know any differently, it is normal for us, until we re-train, re-parent, re-educate ourselves as to what is a healthier way of being. I was, however, in the midst.

I felt constant stress, worry and confusion within me and surrounding me at work. In the early 90's, I became ill with a virus. We are more susceptible to infections when cortisol, the stress hormone, is present continually. I was scared, I had few tools to protect myself with and no assertion techniques, just anger if I blew my top on occasions I felt really pushed. I had no concept of 'boundaries', what on earth were they?! I'd 'freeze'. The fight, flight or freeze response is where in certain situations you feel overpowered. 'Freeze' is often linked to trauma or autistic spectrum tendencies, so I mostly couldn't articulate myself, or occasionally, when really pushed, I would blow my top and tip over into rage.

## All about M.E.

I was given antibiotics, and continued working. By then, I'd been given a sideways move to behavioural science, away from the other colleague. However, one day I just couldn't get up. I went off sick and could not recover from the infection. 'Yuppy flu' it was called back then in the early 90's. Less was known about it then (not that we've progressed much) but as my GP said in a letter to the company doctor at the time 'I believe she has M.E., if you believe in that'. He was a supportive GP towards me, but there was no support because they didn't whether M.E. was real or just 'malingering'. People find it difficult to understand, or believe. With M.E. you can often look so well, but are just left with a lead weight tiredness in the body, and it was too tiring to even make a cup of tea. Coupled with the depression and now changes in Seroxat medication I was taking, I became suicidal. I'd had such thoughts in the past when life was too painful and unbearable, but up until then I'd never acted on those thoughts. There followed, on a number of occasions, a number of suicide attempts. Life was too painful, I couldn't see a way through or out of it. I didn't know how to support myself. I began to even doubt myself, maybe I was just lazy, a malingerer, why couldn't I think my way out of it?

## Deaths and the light of near death

A few years down the line, I'd moved house to North Wales. I was still battling with depression and M.E. Five family members had died within six months, including my Gran who I felt a family connection of 'this is where I come from' with. I often used to feel like I was born into the wrong family. It was a very distressing time, as my Grandad then died six weeks later, of a broken heart. By then I just felt like I wanted to be with my Gran, it was all too much and I wrote letters to everyone saying goodbye.

In unbearable mental pain, I took another overdose. I had a near death experience where I saw a beautiful pure white light, just like magnesium burning and felt a sense of peace which was literally out of this world. It was like nothing I'd ever felt before. I woke up feeling like I was obviously here for a reason, as I'd tried a number of times now to end my life. I just didn't know what that reason was, or why. I wasn't told, I didn't see any angels at that point or any people, I just thought, well I keep trying to end my life, perhaps it's just not going to happen! Ironically, on waking, those of us who have come round after suicide attempts can even feel a sense of failure at not being able to even get that right! So I wondered, maybe there is another way. And rock bottom does sometimes ,by its very nature, show us those ways.

Out of chaos and out of the void, comes the light of creation, something new comes and out of it is born. Like the phoenix rising from the ashes or a baptism of fire, it certainly was! It was a dissolution of the ego and the most painful transformation process. I was convinced that I would be dead by the time I was twenty-five years old and I sometimes marvel that I am still here and got through that terrible time.

## Initiatory experiences

Spiritually and shamanically, such life experiences can be also known as initiations. They open us up to greater things, but at the time it is hell, the belief that we are not going to make it through such pain is the initiation which ultimately transforms and transmutes us. People say that religion is for people who believe in hell and spirituality is for people who have been to hell. It is the death card in the tarot, the point where everything ends so that we can begin anew, just like the winter precedes the spring and new life.

I had no faith, I'd been down on bent knees in my darkness praying that if there was a God 'please help me', but what I was really asking for was a magic wand to take it away there and then. I didn't realise that in fact my prayers were being answered. They can take a while for us to see, feel or hear that.

It's like the story about the guy who is on a desert island and prays to God for help, God sends a ship and the man waves it away saying 'It's ok, I've asked God to help me'. So God sends another ship, and another. The man just doesn't get it. It's that preconceived idea of what help should look like, we get stuck in that, instead of trying out a few options. So the guy dies and says to God when he gets to the otherworld, 'why didn't you help?' to which, of course, God replies 'I did… you just didn't listen'. We then may realise that we have always been guided, it's just that we didn't or couldn't hear!

I'd closed my ears to the God of traditional religion when we went to church as a child. It not only bored me rigid (coupled with low vibes from the cathedral, and our local church, I have never found them to be spiritually light places) but moreso because I sat there one day, aged eight, thinking 'this really is a farce'. It was insisted upon that we come to church on a Sunday, but religion isn't really something that seemed to work in practice. They then treated me and others with condemnation during the week and isn't this the cause of wars? The thoughts of many. There's something not quite right about this.

I did feel that there was something greater than I, when I'd looked up at the stars as a child and got that sense of awe, wasn't that what it was about? There was some force that was awesome and so as I grew older I had just tried to treat others as I would want to be treated myself, to be kind and good in my own way as best I could, but I also made a fair few mistakes myself. I came to realise that life just isn't black and white. And from then a path did start to be forged in the spirit of Self-Care, but it took me a long time to acknowledge or see that I was being led or guided down that path and that my prayers were being answered.

## Animal constants

A major factor in the unfolding of my life coming together was meeting a beautiful little cat called Poppy. It is with many thanks to her little soul that I am sitting here writing a self care book. I will tell you more about that in the animals as rescuers chapter, but suffice to say for now, her and Harriet, my other little cat, had a huge impact on me through their therapeutic wellbeing but also my care of them.

## Finding my passion

I was claiming disability benefits due to my health. I really didn't like being on benefits, I felt very ashamed that I wasn't contributing or paying my way. I always had it as a goal to return to work, but how?

Caring for animals gave me a purpose, life became much more meaningful for me and you can read more about that in the animals and their rescue humans chapter. I was trying to find something meaningful in my life. I began to find my passion, my joy in life and a reason for being. My animal family got me up every day and even if the rest of the day I was lying down tired and rock bottom depressed, they were company for me too.

## Epiphany

My self-care epiphany occurred when I was caring for Poppy. Through that journey it opened up my eyes to what I was not doing for myself. Perhaps I needed to help myself! But how? A few years later a lady came into my life who was also pivotal in helping me. I will be eternally grateful to her for helping me to turn my life around. She was a medium and she somewhat reluctantly explained to me that she thought that some of the issues that I was having were because I was psychic and you will read more of that as the self-care insights unfold.

Over the following years, with her help, I tested out the ability to 'see, hear and feel' on a psychic level, and to learn more about energy therapies such as spiritual healing and Reiki. These were a huge calling for me. My learning is mainly through what is sometimes known as direct revelation. Often I find that I have the experience in life, make sense of it, receive guidance about it through meditation or whilst out running or walking, then read a book which confirms what has just happened. This is enough to reassure me. I've been guided for many years, originally without realising what was going on, as is often the case for some of us on a similar path. Over the years, as I've come to understand more, that my understanding and answers come through omens, synchronicity and direct revelation as I connect with my higher self or soul, God (a kind, loving, non-judgmental God, think 'Conversations with God') angels, spirit guides, nature and animals.

Events conspired to support me in the journey to become the Holistic Therapist that I am today, I trained in Reiki, then went on to do some counselling training and then qualified in holistic therapies to set up my own practise, 'in the heart of the community'. I still struggled with my health, the path of wellness isn't a linear line and there are often backwards and forwards steps. My GP diagnosed fibromyalgia due to the myriad of aches and pains and other symptoms I experienced, and CFS was the rheumatologist's diagnosis some years later, who recommended more holidays! That was motivation enough as I'd started to venture further afield.

Because of these personal experiences and having to take good care of and manage my health so consciously, I recognise just how VITAL* it is to practice self-care, as a therapist. In that way I feel grateful that I have had health problems which have ramped up the necessity for self-care, but opened my eyes in the process. I sincerely believe that the therapeutic community are not given enough training in this area of work because I see how many therapists, who are truly good therapists, could be even better if they were able to practice committed self-care. But we just don't always know how to do so because of our blocks. It's as if we're blind to it and perhaps that's just our different paths anyway. It is said that 'the meaning of life is to find our gift and the purpose of life is to give it away'.

Through that, I hope this book about self-care can help you to find your inner self-carer which strengthens or ignites your own gifts in life!

*Vital means energetic and full of life

# Chapter One

# Helper Heal Thyself

One of my favourite expressions, that repeatedly came into my mind when I started my journey of psychic and spiritual development was 'healer heal thyself'. I realised that I had a lot of work to do on myself and that realisation was a blessing. I intuitively felt that one of my goals in life was to turn my painful experiences into something that would help others. But I couldn't help them until I helped myself. I feel fortunate that the work that I had to do on myself was apparent. If we are functioning pretty well in life, it may be harder to see what work we might need to do on ourselves. I felt so broken, that it seemed like I had to rebuild myself. It was like starting from scratch. This in itself is often seen as an initiation process, or shamanic sickness.

It is also worth bearing in mind that we don't have to be fully 'healed' in order to begin to help others. I'm pretty sure no one who does this work is so and I think we probably wouldn't be here on earth if that were the case! It can frequently be the case that by helping others, we help ourselves. Whilst doing so, it is an astute individual that keeps one eye on their own issues and takes good care of their own needs. On my journey, I soon came to hear about the scenario of the wounded healer and the rescuer, which made a lot of sense.

## The Wounded Healer and the Rescuer

Many people who are drawn to the helping professions, or are givers, may share a common theme which is that of the wounded healer. At some point we may have experienced injustice, suffering or abuse. Pain can open us up. It can follow that we more easily relate with empathy and compassion to another's suffering, their feelings of helplessness or isolation. This can promote in us a strong desire or drive to ease that suffering in others.

However, it can help us to be aware of and to address the possibility of imbalances which can occur within relationships where we may feel the desire, or even a need, to 'fix', 'heal', 'cure' or help others. Do we like to be needed is the first question that we can ask ourselves. Do we feel a thrill, perhaps even a sense of power, when we think that we can be of help to another? What issues do we still have that still require our attention? What do we have difficulty addressing?

However difficult it may be, it may help us to consider that by wanting to help others, we could still be running from our own unhealed wounds. To see another in distress can remind us, all too easily, of our own pain that might yet be unresolved. Rather than confront our own pain, by looking within, it is sometimes easier for us to want to save the world instead. Another of my favourite quotes is by Gandhi, when he said 'We must be the change that we want to see in the world'. The onus for change lies within ourselves. We may want to live in a peaceful world, but how can we demonstrate peace 'fully', if we ourselves lack inner peace?

To be aware of and to know of our own motivations for wanting to help others gives us a firmer foothold along a complex path. If we are still clouded with pain ourselves there can be an unconscious drive of not so self-less motives. Hidden motivations can cause us to place conditions upon another, whether we are aware of those or not. We may still have subconscious expectations which can have a knock-on effect on those that are vulnerable. This can lead us into territory which is unethical and cause more damage to another than good. For example, we may want another person to get better, because it makes us feel like we are doing a good job. The client may feel a subtle pressure, on a subconscious level. If the client doesn't get better, we may feel frustrated with them, which if not addressed in supervision may be felt by the client on a subtle level. That person may start to feel that they are not 'performing' or 'getting it right'. However, if we have our own self-awareness and accept that the journey is different for all of us and takes varying amounts of time, we can side-step the similarities and just hold a space for that person to be as they are - different to us.

It is good self-care to commit to regular therapies, therapy and/or supervision, when we know that we still have unresolved issues that cause us problems. That would probably mean everyone, because who doesn't on some level or other! An inability to address our own inner pain with courage, clarity and compassion is the greatest irony of the helping and healing professions.

As helpers and givers, we may not be walking our talk in the path of the truth that we believe if we are encouraging others to have help, yet aren't open to that ourselves. 'Do as I say, not as I do' sends out mixed messages. If we lack authenticity and genuineness, on some level, that conflict can be perceived by others. I often get asked who I go to for therapy. Admission of our own vulnerabilities and our imperfections, and practising trust of others by sharing these qualities in appropriate circumstances can ultimately build up our own trust in our Self and our sense of self-worth.

As a giver or therapist, it's OK to be less than perfect; it's grounding to be less than perfect when we own those qualities. It can be quite a relief, instead of burying our shadow aspects and glossing over our truth with a shiny persona of how perfect we and our lives are. The admission of 'just as we are' can open up honest communication, trust and understanding with others. I've noticed how it often promotes liberation in others too, when one person in a group admits to their vulnerabilities. It's so much easier once we have taken steps to admit our truth. This sharing with appropriate people, can be healing in itself if this is the approach that you choose to use.

## The Butterfly

When I am in a place of feeling like I am drawn into someone's story, yet something is also holding me back from it and the toxic guilt threatens to overspill, I endeavour to remind myself of the following. I have seen this many times in action. It is ironic that we think that rescuing other people helps them, when sometimes it really can be to their detriment. It seems contrary to everything that we have learnt and are told in our co-dependant society. 'Help, I need somebody!'

More people are waking up to the truth that our inner self becomes stronger when we help ourselves. This involves maintaining a compassionate space for others, rather than coldly saying, 'get on with it' or putting a barrier up (as I have done myself at times). It's about stepping back, with love and compassion, for what that person is going through. Sometimes this is easier to do in a professional capacity because there are firmer boundaries in place that prevent us from getting overly involved. When I have stepped back, much to the person's chagrin at times (but with very firm inner guidance and gut feeling on occasions), that person really has flourished, because they have had to learn to do something by themselves. Helping them would have taken that experience away.

Out walking, I saw a young lad and his mum, seated on a wide bench. The young lad was trying to crawl up onto his mum's shoulders and she was encouraging him to do so. In busy body fusspot mode, I could have gone over and helped him, as I was tempted to do. But what would he have gained? Nothing much. Instead I would have stolen his sense of achievement when he did it by himself. It's a kind of energy theft. I myself would have felt better in that moment, but long term he'd have lost out. Sometimes I find that if I truly believe in someone's ability, just telling them that when they are struggling, as I have been told myself, can be very empowering and touching. When I have to step back, I remind myself of the following story that was doing the email rounds some years ago.

"A man came across a cocoon of a butterfly. A small opening appeared in the cocoon one day and the man watched the struggle of the butterfly for some hours as it tried to emerge from the tiny hole. It then appeared to stop making progress, that it had got as far as it could. The man in his kindness decided to help the butterfly and taking some scissors, cut the cocoon, so that the butterfly could then emerge easily.

The butterfly's body was swollen and it had small shrivelled wings. The man thought that at any moment the wings would unfold and get larger in order to support the butterfly's body. He thought perhaps the butterfly's body might get smaller in time. However, neither of these things happened and the butterfly spent its life crawling round with an enlarged body and shrivelled wings, never able to fly.

The man did not, in his kindness, understand that the restriction of the cocoon and the struggle to emerge, were nature's way of forcing fluid from the body of the butterfly into the wings. This would enable it to be ready for flight once it achieved its release from the cocoon.

Sometimes we need to struggle to grow. If we were to go through our lives with no obstacles it could cripple and disable us. We would not be as strong as we could potentially have been – we would never learn to fly! Something which is always worth bearing in mind with clients too if they are going through a tough time; it may be difficult to watch, but to grow they must come through it themselves. All we can do is hold the space, watch over the process and perhaps if appropriate say a prayer."(Author unknown)

## Accepting we have needs too

Acceptance is an early first hurdle or obstacle that we benefit from overcoming in the process of self-care. Accepting that we too need self-care as a giver and a doer, that we aren't a bottomless source of energy can sometimes be forced upon us when we become chronically ill, or have to stop work due to illness or something else. It can hit us like a kick in the teeth when we realise that we aren't invincible. This can be the gift or the message behind the experience, but certainly doesn't feel like that at the time.

Yet how many of us find that it takes until we get to that point to realise this? I think people will begin to change their perspective as the concept of SC is now becoming more popular, even coining the phrase with memes about 'Self-Care Sunday'. Unfortunately our egos or pride may be an obstacle here, disallowing us the chance to accept help, 'I've got this, I can do it', 'Go me!', 'Strong man/woman!' all designed to block help, reciprocity and deeper healing which allows us to recharge.

## Opening ourselves up to receiving

Allowing ourselves to receive is difficult if we have been used to being the one that is giving. However, that can also commonly be a form of control, where we may think that we know best or don't want to let another person in. Even receiving a compliment can be hard for many, instead of saying 'thank you'. It can be hard to not dismiss a compliment by minimising it, such as when someone says our hair looks nice. Instead we can point out all the faults that we don't like about our hair generally.

One way that I began to allow myself to receive compliments and appreciate them was by realising that I genuinely enjoy complimenting people, if I believe it to be the truth. However some people won't accept a compliment by saying, 'Oh they're just saying that'. I accept that some people do use flattery as a form of manipulation, however, I think many of us can be genuine with our energy, in that way.

When we begin to tune into our own feelings (instead of cutting them off and living in our heads, instead of fully in our bodies), I think we get a sense of when someone is genuine or if they 'just want something'. When they do, it often feels either over the top and excessive adoration and praise if they are being manipulative, or empty of thought or feeling. I reasoned that I like to see people enjoy receiving a compliment, it can sometimes make someone's day to feel noticed and valued, I realised that if I rejected compliments myself I was denying someone the pleasure of seeing me pleased with their compliment. It was in effect dismissing them. This is a first step in learning to receive.

## Can you.. and thank you

Offerings of help, instead of the 'I'll do this' mindset, can help to prevent burn-out. Practising saying thanks might be a little difficult initially, it can be uncomfortable and may even bring up feelings of guilt or shame. Eating a slice of humble pie and realising that there really isn't any shame in not being able or not even wanting to do all and everything and asking for and accepting help is ok. Delegating responsibility, or asking others for help allows us to accept and receive the help that we all need from time to time. Team work isn't a failing!

Realising then that by topping our battery levels up by allowing ourselves to take time for ourselves and doing something for ourselves or having a treatment or allowing someone to treat us, is not a shameful thing. It is only 'a shame' when we cannot say yes and allow. To be so closed to help is quite tragic. If you do nothing else for a month, learn to say yes or thank you at least once a week.

## 'I owe them' mentality

Fear of saying yes might be because you then feel that you owe the other person something. 'One good turn deserves another' can sometimes be used as a lever and they may call in the favour and you don't have the energy to return it. Again another reason why self-care and topping up your batteries is a necessity. I was recently in a similar situation and hadn't felt able for various reasons to go and feed a friend's cat when she had asked. I decided to pay someone, and a figure intuitively came in my head. I asked my friend first and said I was prepared to pay, and in that way didn't have that concern about reciprocal return, as I wasn't feeling up to returning favours. I was also showing her that I valued her time and petrol.

Sometimes, as has been the case for me too, we might not be able to afford to pay someone. It might be that if we are surrounded by people who believe that every kind thing that they do for us needs to be repaid - 'I've done this or that for you'and bring this up regularly, that this is emotional blackmail and a barter system rather than a genuine friendship. It's about needs getting met and possibly time to find true friends, which is also a journey of self-care.

## Give time to yourself

Accepting and allowing, instead of putting up barriers can be hard to overcome, it may be a replay of interpersonal scenarios from the past that trigger those thoughts, rather than there being foundation for them in the present. Such thoughts and the awkwardness can be overcome over time, but it does take time. And that is where we can cultivate patience with ourselves and give ourselves time.

It might be that we also need to accept ourselves for how we are right now. We might be aware that we are unfit and appreciate that we would benefit from going out for a run in the morning, but for some reason, despite our best intentions, it's just not happening. Sometimes I think that we need time for ideas to germinate and come into being. Another of the sayings that often comes through when I do readings is that the fruit needs time to ripen, just as the seed of an idea needs time to germinate.

Sometimes our intuition is indicating to us what is up ahead, so that idea of going out for a run is that seed, it's emerging in our awareness or consciousness and it is coming up, but not right now. We've not got to the green light yet. In the 'mean' time we might be bullying ourselves and berating ourselves harshly for not being able to achieve our goals, when really we aren't even at the starting block! Although we may have intuitions or ideas of what is up ahead, we might not always be given the route or the fine details of the plan. When we give ourselves time, we can literally 'watch this space', that's when the miracle of germination, that positive force of creation, happens. Ideas are born and begin to bear fruit.

## Don't push the river

This was a phrase that came through during a reading, which ultimately says it is pointless or fruitless to try to push the river back upstream. Imagine the scenario; there we are with our bare hands trying to push this cascade of water back upstream. Yet when we are in such a mindset, often we do not take care of ourselves and attempt to do just that, with stubbornness, trying over and over again. Deep inside we know it is probably fruitless. From time to time, granted we may need to overcome the odds and make efforts and during each instance only you can decide that. See also the section on challenging negative thoughts. For me, if I keep experiencing obstacles and I don't have the right tools, it might be that I back off and accept that the current is flowing as it is and the timing is not right, right now.

## Surrendering

Accepting, allowing and letting go is a form of 'surrender'. This doesn't mean that we give up on what we are doing or that we don't take responsibility for it. Surrender, however, can be an effective form of (spiritual) practise and can be quite a relief. Instead of 'giving up' it acknowledges, just like the Serenity Prayer that there are some things in life that we can't control. 'Our way' might not necessarily be the best way, there may be another way which will emerge if we let go of trying so hard. Sometimes we can just do no more, we may think 'that's it, enough, I'm finished, I've tried my best' we've done all we possible can within our means and have to leave the outcome to the powers that be.

For months I was at a stumbling block with decorating the bedroom, I'd chosen the bedding but couldn't decide on the wallpaper. I usually like to put the bedding on when the room is finished, like the icing on the cake. However, my intuition said 'put the bedding on now, get a feel for it'. I surrendered 'my way' (my ego) and within a week I'd decided on the wallpaper and it's the most beautiful bedroom I've ever had!

There is a fierceness of trying too hard, a 'force' of determination that comes from a place of fear and ego, (rather than one of love trust and acceptance). When we let go and surrender and give that up, we energetically create space, we create a void. There is a saying that the universe hates a void, and so what it does is fill the space. Giving up our control and saying to the powers that be or the universal flow, 'show me another way' can allow things to happen, it creates a more fertile space.

Being self-employed can be scary when we know that we need a certain amount of clients to pay the bills. Having that stress upon us, can potentially take some of the passion and enjoyment out of the job. I was given a carved wooden footprint with a fish on it, years ago on a retreat. It had been made by one of the retreat leaders for all of us attending. It was to represent the story in the bible where Jesus turned 5 loaves and 2 fishes into food to feed 5,000. So over the years, that fish has sat on my desk, to remind me that there is enough and have myself gone through phases where I have felt more able to trust the process or the journey than others and the times where I flail, I am carried by that footprint and supported.

I often used to wake up worrying that certain bills needed to be met and my diary was empty. However, something would always come through and happen in the 7th hour. So just when I needed to pay something or other, someone would book in and that bill would be covered. This has happened so frequently since I have been doing this work, that I now have a deeper sense of trust that everything will be OK, there is enough to go round. When I wasn't so trusting, I would often try too hard. I'd frequently send out texts doing special offers, I'd put posts on Facebook with the intention of gaining custom. Whilst is it good to stay visible to clients to remind them you're still in business, I was at times doing this more out of fear of 'not enough' rather than there's availability if you want it, but otherwise I'll just get on with my admin - or my book on self-care! The times I tried out of fear, I'd notice that often I would get no response. I soon came to realise, don't push the river.

Now, I listen for intuitive nudges if I'm to post on Facebook or send out a text with a special offer. I don't do it out of fear. And I allow the powers that be to plan my diary, I love this! It might be that the gaps in my diary allow me to do other things such as admin that I might have to do at home if I was otherwise full. I also used to set a target goal of how much money I would need, for example if I was going away.

However, I also came to realise that what is available is always the perfect amount. My role of responsibility is to listen to the intuitive nudges that I may get about when to take action, rather than thinking I am the be all and end all of the action all the time! That way we go with the flow and can also serve ourselves and others better by this, it's much more relaxed.

Yesterday I had a text from a client who wanted to bring her appointment forward, there was a gap in my diary which allowed her to do that, she was really appreciative. If I'd gone into panic mode that the slots weren't full and advertised, and someone had filled it, her day wouldn't have flowed so well.. and mine - well, I needed the extra time in my diary to pack for coming away to write this. So it all works out perfectly.

Experiment with dropping the belief that you have to do everything yourself and you are the be all and end all. This isn't to disempower you, but quite the opposite, when we work with the flow of the universe, we can often notice that a surge of energy comes to us or wells within us, which is our recharge, our power. We can hand over the reins to the Powers that be who have a much bigger overall picture than we do, and become more effective and less stressed out. As Deepak Chopra calls it 'it's the law of least effort'

## It is, as it is…

We may go through hard tough, times and that is life, accepting that we do and that life can be very hard can allow us to let that energy flow again. If we deny what is happening by saying 'I don't want things to be this way.. I wish they were different', we use up a lot of energy trying to change a reality that sometimes is as it is. Sometimes we are powerless. We can do no more. Saying 'I wish the lights were on green', won't make them change. Sitting patiently knowing that they are on red and accepting that is energy conservation, because it is as it is! Even better when we put the intention out there that we'd like to get through the lights quickly, but accept that if someone else's need is greater, that they go first.

## Avoiding disaster…

Besides which, with the overseeing powers that be, I sometimes wonder if I am late because I've got caught in an unexpected jam, or as happened recently there are road blocks up ahead. There could be something down the road that I might be best avoiding. If I am running a bit later, it may be for what I believe is 'my highest good', or the good of my soul or self. We may actually avoid catastrophe on the road ahead, by being later.

## Let go and let the powers that be…

One of my difficulties, being a bit of an ex-perfectionist, is wanting to 'make sure that I include everything that I know that can help another in this book'. This attitude creates a stress immediately, as I can't give others all of their answers, neither remember all of the experiences that have got me thus far! Accepting that I bring through what is needed for this book and that is enough, will help me to complete it. In the past I have put myself under pressure to be the be all and end all which is depleting of the creative flow. I've surrendered the contents and the process up to the powers that be, I step aside and become the channel for that. In Reiki, we do similar. We step aside and let the energy flow through us, we are just an empty vessel and 'let go and let God', we get our ego out of the way of the process (sometimes also known as hollowing out).

## Letting people down

I had another wake up call today about another block that I have with self-care. I was awake in the night for some hours having woken up nauseous; I'd caught a minor sickness bug that my partner had a few days prior. When it came time to get up, I still felt ill. It was a cold, icy, frosty morning, I had nearly an hours drive for therapy and I didn't feel well enough. Several things came up for me as I was challenging myself to push through it or not, because I knew it had passed quickly for my partner. One thing that crossed my mind was it would pass quickly if I gave myself a push, and in general it was bringing up thoughts of discomfort about 'letting others' down', not being enough, etc. I knew, on one level, that this was not letting my counsellor down, I didn't want to pass it on to her either; yet it was echoing that memory that many of us have which causes us to push through times when we don't feel up to it, because we don't want to let others down or disappoint them. This may be telling of our own disappointment and it may help us to look at times when we have felt let down ourselves. Can you recall any time that you have felt let down and can you allow yourself to feel that disappoint?

## Default mechanisms

There was also an overhang from being chronically ill. Many who are or have been often won't be or feel able to attend all commitments, despite wanting to. As I reflected on this, I realised that also, for years, not knowing what the feeling of being well was, I was in a perpetual habit of having to push myself. It was default mechanism to survive. So whereas someone who's health comes and goes will then perhaps be able to say I'm well I'll go to do xyz, someone with chronic illness may be like a stuck record, stuck in that place of pushing. Returning to well-being and then knowing the difference that this is a different sort of illness and it's ok to have some down time can take a bit of re-educating and it can take time to change that habit. Pushing ourselves through illness and living with chronic illness can be 'normal', you just learn to get on and live with it, which can really skew the concept of self-care and the point at which you stop and have that down-time. On the flip-side of that is that this can be the causes of illness becoming more and more chronic, as we don't know how to switch off.

# Chapter Two

## How Selfish to Burnout!

### Self care and why you might need it

Burnout, or compassion fatigue, is common among among the helping professions such as social workers, counsellors, support workers and care staff, doctors, nurses, police, carers (particularly unpaid) and holistic therapists. Other professions such as charity workers and in particular the teaching professions can be vulnerable to stress and the risk of burnout; teaching is on the top level of 'stressful' occupations, when I ask clients what they do. As well as parents. Mothers will often say that because they put themselves to one side to meet the needs of their children, in doing so they have lost their sense of identity. Becoming consumed with that role of 'Mother' they may wonder years later, when their children leave home, who they really are as a person, because they've invested so much of themselves in their children. Particularly parents who have children with special needs will probably feel the pull of exhaustion and burnout if they don't have adequate support.

What is probably common to all of these people is that they have an openness and desire to help others, possibly because of their own life experiences which have touched them. They are all Givers with a capital G and probably perfectionists too, where they give not just 100%, but 120%. It often isn't until someone falls chronically ill, or goes off work with stress that they become aware of what is often called 'burnout'. When we understand a little more of the signs of that and how it affects us, we can guard against it.

Allowing ourselves to rest if we are a giver and a doer may seem a nigh on impossible task, as it may feel like we are the only person who can do it all and feel overly responsible. There can be a myriad of other reasons why we can't allow ourselves to 'just be' and to receive help ourselves. Burnout is the phone that hasn't been recharged, and has gone flat; it's power has gone, but knowing how to effectively plug in and recharge for us as an individual is what counts - remember different phones have different chargers and it's finding the right charger for you as a person!

## Symptoms of Burnout

### Irritability
We may find that we develop an intolerance towards other people, which isn't normal for us. Feelings of anger, frustration and disdain may creep in.

### Lack of empathy
Whereas previously we may have had bucket loads of compassion and empathy for the plight or circumstances of others, it may feel like we don't just don't care anymore or don't have it in us to care. If we are in a helping profession we may begin to dislike our job, or our children, becoming resentful of their needs. We can't serve from that empty cup. Instead we may feel that we want to distance ourselves from others and the last thing that we may want to do is socialise, we may just not have the energy.

### Mental and emotional symptoms
Switching off mentally may be a real challenge, it can feel like our brain is always on the go, at 20, 000 mile per hour! Taking work home can creep up on us, until we realise that we are thinking about clients or what we have to do the next day and

those thoughts of work are excessive and may wake us at night.

Our mental processes may begin to suffer where we are so tired we literally can't think or process things properly. Our memory may start to suffer, where we find recall of events or details difficult and lack focus or concentration (brain fog). Not being able to even think about the simple things and finding that we don't even care anymore, 'I've had it!'may be a proclamation as we go into shutdown.

Waking up depressed with a more negative outlook on life than before and feelings of doom may feature. This is as if something bad is going to happen and a sense of being on edge all the time; not being able to relax properly. We may experience anxiety and even panic attacks and begin to catastrophise, thinking about worse case scenarios of what might go wrong in the future. Watching TV or a film, or interacting with others we can notice that we're crying more frequently or at 'little' things and not really know why. There may be a feeling of being more permeable, vulnerable and defenceless.

Procrastination may become a factor if we find that we are de-motivated. Waking in the morning and not wanting to go to work or not getting work done by putting it off, or experiencing a lack of concentration. It could be that we are then overly critical of ourselves for not achieving our goals, particularly if we have perfectionistic tendencies. With a cynical attitude and the passion and drive for what we care about depleted, we may find ourselves thinking 'what's the point in doing this?'

A sense of frustration and powerlessness can often accompany burnout if for instance the organisation that we work for do not support self-care or sufficiently value their staff. It can be quite common to hear of support workers who are covering hours for others, because the organisation just can't get the staff. I often think about the irony of the NHS for example, on the whole they are caring workers trying to do the best they can, with the resources that they have, but the foundation for the staff support seems to be lacking and in that way not healthy, but quite 'sick'. I asked a client, who is a nurse, during a consultation, whether she drank enough water and she laughed and said no, she worked for the NHS! She's overworked and doesn't get chance to have a drink, but she loves her job.

**Feeling trapped - there's no way out!**
Putting our bodies under continual stress like that will not help the battery levels and eventually can cause problems. However sometimes we can feel trapped - 'it's a job after all'. With bills to pay it can seem like we have little choice until that choice seems to be made for us, through the wake up call of ill health. Charitable organisations also are renowned 'takers' of their workers by their very nature, attracting unpaid workers who at first are happy and more than willing to give extra hours because of their kind natures and passion for great causes. Sometimes there is guilt to overwork because they see that's what volunteers and other workers are doing too. Learning to put boundaries in place, drop the toxic guilt and realise that we are doing a good enough job, are all measures that we may need to put in place to prevent our energy leakages!

As an attempt to quell the difficulty of managing burnout some people find that they turn to crutches such as food or drink to ease or comfort themselves. Others may lose their appetite and lose weight, finding the thought of food makes them feel nauseous.

## Physical Exhaustion & Disrupted Sleep

Feeling more tired than usual, fatigued or chronic fatigue (waking feeling exhausted and unrefreshed from sleep) may kick in on a physical level. We may not have the energy to move our body in the way that we have before. It can feel like we are carrying a lead weight around with us. Do check with your GP if you have experience these symptoms for any length of time.

Despite feeling exhausted, our sleep cycle can get disrupted. We may wake frequently at night, churning thoughts over, or worrying and have long period of being wide awake and not being able to fall back to sleep. Feeling exhausted during the day due to lack of good quality sleep at night, an afternoon nap might seem desirable - yet then cause us not to sleep so well that night.

## Susceptibility to illness and physical symptoms

When we are burning out or burnt out, our susceptibility to infections, viruses, colds and flu increases. Illnesses such as coughs can take longer to recover from. When I was suffering from M.E. I couldn't understand how anyone could 'just' have a cold. If I caught one I'd often be in bed for two weeks, it would always go onto my chest (smoking didn't help). As my health improved and my battery recharged, it was wonderful to just have a 'normal' cold where my energy levels didn't feel completely depleted and I could, go down a gear, but mostly carry on with my day.

Digestive problems due to stress, such as Irritable Bowel Syndrome (IBS) can be accompanied by anxious churning feelings in the stomach. It might be that we have been in fight or flight mode for too long, if stress has been a factor for a while. We may have nausea, acid reflux and intermittent constipation or diarrhoea. Again, please check out symptoms with a GP for any underlying conditions. A physical illness may cause symptoms which make you feel more stressed - which you might otherwise cope with, so it might be an illness, not burnout.

All sorts of physical symptoms, often in the form of aches and pains, can arise. When we experience the mental and emotional symptoms of tension, and don't know how to diffuse these or discharge them, it can frequently be transferred to the body as tension. Think about someone who is tense and how they may hold their fist tightly. That tension then goes all the way up the arm to the shoulders, or they may sit with their shoulders hunched and rounded in a defeated or defensiveness position. This tension can lead to all sorts of other physical aches and pains: jaw clenching, bad back or the necks are particular areas of the body, as well as the scalp and even the feet.

## So what are our blocks to self-care?

Our resistance and our blocks to self-care can deplete us, rather than allow us to recharge. This could be likened to the apps that run in the background of our phone and computer; they are not featuring or observable on the main screen (within our consciousness and awareness), but they are still there working in the background which ultimately depletes our energy. We need to learn to switch those apps off so they stop working randomly or willy nilly and depleting the battery. We need to optimise ourselves! With awareness that those apps are there and perhaps why they are, we can overcome our barriers to self-care. What we can ask ourselves in these scenarios and once we become familiar with the apps that are running in our own background and what is draining us is - can I afford to do this? What is the physical, mental, emotional and energetic cost to me if I neglect my own self-care needs? That awareness can suffice to get us through those mindful moments of self-neglect, and once we arm ourselves with a variety of battery chargers, we may find that we can replenish ourselves on fast charge anyway, because we've come to understand what works for us.

## So what are your blocks to self-care and what challenges you?

'I can't put myself first, it's selfish, I feel mean!' This is probably the most common stumbling block for allowing ourselves to receive or give or care for ourselves. It can feel alien, very odd to think of ourselves in receipt of something if we are natural givers. It may be that all of our lives we have given and done for others, perhaps because that was what was expected of us and it became part of our persona or identity. Giving to others can be deeply ingrained and habitual. It can also be part of our survival strategy in childhood, that if we please the parent or guardian, it will ensure that at least some of our needs are met.

So how did we come to be like that? During the course of this book, we will look at those obstacles and the programmes that go on within us. Some of these are unconscious and out of our awareness, until someone or something brings them to light. Sometimes it may only be when we are so ill that we have to play detective to find out what went wrong, in order to rectify our health.

With this in mind, this book might be triggering. It could open things up for you. Some of the scenarios may bring back painful memories for you. If so, do the self-care and seek help from a trained therapist who understands your situation, for support. It is likely if you are reading this book, that you need some help with self care as it doesn't, or hasn't, come naturally to you. Me too, as you may have read in the foreword. Hence why and how I write this. As I often say to my clients, I've worn and continue to wear the t-shirt! I've made many mistakes which means I can sit there and say yes it can be really tough, but there are little things you can do that help. Being more aware of what your obstacles are can help raise that awareness which really can turn your life around, as it has mine.

## There are reasons

Not really thinking about what we want or need to do and paying attention to that can mean that we become like robots on automation as our lives become emptier of 'us' and more about others. Through that, life can lose its true meaning. If we have people around us who don't take no for an answer and have strategies to ensure that they get what they want at a cost to us, we may appease them 'just for a quiet life'. We may feel bad if we say no, guilty, mean, powerless as if we have no choice, despairing and fearful of consequences. There may be many other conflicting feelings that get in the way of us taking better care of ourselves and preventing burn out. We may just love giving to others, it's part of who we are, it's a joy for us and does give our life meaning.

## 2. How Selfish to Burn Out

It is important to notice and remember as you read through this book, that there are often reasons why we do or don't do things. Our ego, or our persona, which is the part of us which often tries to keep us safe, or get us through life, is constructed in the way that it is and shouldn't be judged for doing so. We have all done the job of life so far, as best we can, to the best of our ability (even if that includes some so called negative aspects and experiences).

Our behaviours change from childhood as a result of the feedback that we get from our family, our environment and society. As youngsters we are dependent on others to get our needs met such as food, shelter, clothing and protection. Our goal is to grow, to meet those innate needs that we have. We adapt to the circumstances that we are in, in response to what pleases or is acceptable to those who will meet our needs.

This 'creates' the persona, the part of us that we present to the world, and perhaps also to ourselves. Because we are social beings, there is strength in numbers and we also have a craving for love to sustain our emotional wellbeing. We aren't always aware that we have, or still are, sacrificing parts of ourselves to literally fit in. Underneath we may have a burning rage that we have been deprived, but because we know the potentiality and consequences of that deprivation, we may put a brave face on in order to get fed. Hence we may become a people pleaser as we push that rage down and put a smile on our face.

We may still be aware of the rage that is suppressed, or we may have kept it hidden away 'in a box' out of our own awareness. Sometimes this is known as the 'shadow'. Often the shadow are seen as the parts of us that are undesirable characteristics or traits, such as greed or laziness. As an adult, if we are aware of them, it might be that we feel that we still need to keep these aspects hidden, because we are judging ourselves unfairly for them. So as adults we repeat that cycle that kept them hidden. After all, who would want to talk to a counsellor who is angry, or see a holistic therapist who is so judgemental and critical of others, we may say to ourselves and in order to do that job, it continues to be hidden.

However, by sacrificing those parts of ourselves unconsciously, and because it is often out of our awareness, particularly as young children, we might not be conscious of those hidden aspects. We may also be denying our true selves or our inherent nature. When we get stressed or tired, or burnt out, it is then that those aspects can leak out and we find we can't control them, 'we lose it'. Those parts are often waving their hand for attention and nourishment themselves and a big dose of healthy compassion. Telling someone that they are bad for being angry doesn't stop the anger, it just pushes it inwards again. Accepting the anger, not judging it, and using various methods such as in shadow work or counselling to give this part of us a voice, may help to dissipate it.

So we have done well to create these strategies that have got us through. We are who we are and where we are, because we've done the best we can with what we have. Now, though, it might be time to change them. As you go through this book, please remember to give yourself that big healthy dose of compassion, if you can't change or understand something right now, it might not be your way. Be kind to you, be your own best friend. I love the words from Max Ehrmans Desiderata, 'beyond a wholesome discipline, be gentle with yourself. You are a child of the universe, no less than the trees and the stars; you have a right to be here'

## But it's selfish!

I muse upon how this feeling of taking care or doing something for ourselves is often blocked by ourselves, or sometimes another, by saying that we are 'being selfish'. If we are told that this is the case by another it may serve us well to bear in mind that this could be a potentially manipulative statement on their part. It could be that they themselves are selfish and want something, 'selfishly from us'. It may demonstrate a lack of empathy on their part if they have called us selfish, because we cannot meet their needs in that moment.

For example, we may be feeling under the weather and want to rest when a friend turns up needing a lift into town as they are going out and can't drive. That friend may be of the 'all about me' kind, who is self-absorbed, only turns up when she wants something, has a sense of self-importance and entitlement, frequently caught up in some drama or other and doesn't tend to take no for an answer. When the request for a lift comes in, we may say, 'I'm not feeling too well, can you get the bus instead?', the friend wanting her needs met pouts and counteracts us with 'oh don't be so selfish! I've got to meet my boyfriend in 10 minutes and I've just missed the bus'. This is called projection, where someone lacks their own self-awareness of their faults (or good points) and attributes those qualities to another. We look at this a little more in the section on shadow work.

Assuming that it isn't 'burn out', if we have been told frequently or repeatedly that we are selfish, there are two option's to consider. We may be surrounded by people who are manipulative and use emotional blackmail to get what they want from us by using it as a lever. We may then begin to take it on board that we are selfish, maybe they are right? Rather than questioning that it might be the friend's own selfishness for not considering that we feel under the weather, we may start to believe that we are the selfish one, especially if we keep attracting selfish people into our lives who call us that and dump it on us! Would you do that to a friend, if they were under the weather? Likely not! Who is the selfish person? The other consideration is, that it could be a shadow aspect of ourselves, as we go into later, and that we are being selfish in that moment. We can all be at times and maybe that is OK sometimes too.

## Don't take it on board!

So when we understand about projection, when someone is trying to dump their stuff on us by saying, 'you're so selfish!'. We may have a thought process of 'oh my goodness am I? Perhaps I am!.. oh hang on a minute, what's that projection thing, maybe they are talking about themselves!' Go off and ask another reliable trustworthy source, a friend who is fair-minded and honest, to check out the validity of that statement, so that you don't take their stuff on board.

## Are you indeed selfish?

In another scenario, feeling under the weather as before, your young child suddenly cries out in pain and deathly white clutches her tummy and vomits. To not pay attention to her needs would at that point would certainly be selfish (as well as neglectful), your gut feeling says she needs to go to the doctor, but you don't because you want to stay home and have a bottle of wine with your friend who is coming round tonight. You'll see how she is in the morning.

## 2. How Selfish to Burn Out

As I said previously, I doubt someone who is reading this sort of book is truly selfish. However, as I've also said, don't we all have times when we are and we can be selfish? Are you ever truly unconditional? We are human after all, we're not perfect. Perhaps just by acknowledging that 'yes at times I can be selfish' and not judge ourselves for it, even accepting that trait, can be quite liberating too (and also may stop us being manipulated). When we own our shadow or dark aspects and accept them, they don't rear their ugly heads at unexpected moments or during times of stress. We can observe them in a detached way and just think, 'oh there goes my selfish part again. I quite fancy doing this and I don't want to help you today'... other times it might be that inner nudge that says you really do need to recharge, 'so yes today I need to do this for me, so I will get Melfish!'

# Chapter Three

## Valuing ourselves

### Value - financial and otherwise

Value is often reflected by society in financial terms. Holistically I see money as a form of material, grounded 'energy'. Money gets us from A to B in the 'real' world that we live in so that we and others can function better. What we purchase has financial value and what we get paid, or charge another for what we do, also has a value. Besides the financial grounded aspects of 'value', there is the value and appreciation for the qualities that we see in ourselves or in another and our gratitude for that - or our disregard. There is also the value for the essence of life itself in spiritual terms and how we may cherish ourselves or one another. Value has far reaching implications and touches on many elements of our lives.

It's often said. 'Do we value our time?' Those that have an abundance of time may not appreciate fully how valuable that time might be to someone who doesn't have it. In similar terms the millionaire whose financial abundance enables them to easily afford the small things in life that others may revere. I remember the feeling of having made it when I could afford to buy screen wash that didn't freeze in winter from the shop, instead of using washing up liquid!

These are generalisations to illustrate the concept of material and financial value, as well as valuing ourselves, noticing our self-worth and how interlinked it can all be. For instance, appreciating that those qualities of kindness and empathy that are natural to us can be of real value therapeutically and when we have sufficient regard for ourselves, the renumeration for that and a job well done helping another can lead to a fortuitous life for all concerned! Win, win!

Part of valuing, in my understanding, is that it is a flow of energy that keeps going. At work, when I charge another for what I do, I can then use that to pay someone else to do what they do. But value goes so much deeper than financial transactions on a material physical level, so deeply that we are often not aware of the roots of why we may find it difficult to charge others for our services or even value ourselves enough to brush our teeth in the morning. The consequences of not valuing ourselves are far reaching.

## Echo supplies Narcissus, but not herself

Narcissus is the character in Greek mythology who fell in love with his own reflection when he saw himself in the water. Echo fell in love with Narcissus. Echo could only repeat the words of others and so mirrored Narcissus, which illustrates a typical co-dependant relationship. I often wonder if this is how many therapists and counsellors 'are born', or 'trained' if one or other of their parents are narcissistic on some level or other. It does seem a common finding for part of the journey of personal development to become aware of that. It is also worth mentioning that we can all have narcissistic traits and if you are wondering whether you are a narcissist too, you probably aren't, as most of them wouldn't even consider themselves to be anything less than perfect. Sadly it's too painful for them to attain that self-awareness, the fallout of not doing so wreaks havoc on those around them.

Narcissus is 'self-absorbed' and Echo is 'other-absorbed'. To break the spell, Echo would benefit from the balance of noticing her own reflection and what is going on for her, but sadly that never happens in the story and she wastes away pining (characteristically dying of self-neglect). Interestingly with the mirroring process of Echo, and the journey of someone who is highly empathic, empathy has been found to be linked with an excess of mirror neurons in the brain. There is a physiological foundation for the way that Echo is too, which invites the nature nurture debate! My money (or value!) is on the nurture aspect being a significant part of Echo's moulding.

A skewed sense of self-value, how we are valued by others and expectations of that process, may come from having had a damaging relationship with a narcissist, either whilst growing up or as an adult. A narcissist's behaviour can be overt or covert. They are characteristically self-absorbed and excessively admire themselves, with an inflated sense of self-importance. They have a lack of heartfelt interest or genuine empathy for others and they have a deep need for lavish attention and praise. Commonly known as narcissistic supply, a narcissist will value another based on what they can get from them. If their association with you brings them attention or kudos, 'you're in'. It's very similar to the playground scenario (that also plays out in adulthood) where someone is 'using you' for what they can get. It's also similar to what people do when they are name-dropping, they are taking the energy from that person's 'name', their 'power', in order to attain that attention for themselves, rather than generating the energy from themselves. It's a form of energy theft which can leave people feeling bereft and empty.

A narcissist will speak to others about you, to impress and gain attention from them, but are unlikely to praise you directly, apart from the early 'love-bombing' stages in a relationship. The narcissist's target or prey (they are predatory, they home in) becomes an object for the narcissist to 'make them look good' in the eyes of others. Think of the typical ambitious stage school mother who pushes the child who has no interest.

'Beryl from the club', is another example, who may haughtily announce to her friends 'my daughter Cassandra has just climbed Everest and been on the front page of National Geographic for her world renowned botany study in Borneo. Whilst on the plane there she sat next to the Prince of Timbuktu who wants her to come and ride his horses as she's such an accomplished dressage rider'. Poor Cassandra, everyone gets bored of hearing about her. It can border on ridiculous sometimes, but does belie a more sinister twist, when we look at the impact that this has on those around them. Cassandra is probably doing all she can to achieve, in the vain hope that she will gain some genuine love and affection for her true self from her mother. Then finally her mum will love her for who she is and tell her that and all will be well in the world. Ultimately Cassandra may find that she needs to pay attention and love to herself to find out who she really is. And put some strong boundaries with Beryl in place too.

Noticing that interest has peaked in the narcissist, if there is something of value to be shared with others, (that will gain some attention for themselves), it can leave those that have been around narcissists not feeling truly loved for who they are, but for what they do. The targeted person may be left with a skewed sense of the expectations of others and what their own values are in life. On the plus side of that, it probably also means that someone who has been in that situation is very able and equipped to deliver and meet another's needs with exceptional acuity and often empathy. Plus a lot of self-care work to make up for the lack of genuine love.

## Disregard and disrespect

A lack of self-value can lead us to be disregarded by others and disrespected. If we send out a message that we don't really care about ourselves, what a huge thing to say - if not verbally then energetically! I do believe that people respond to energy subconsciously; consider the 'hen pecking'scenario mentioned in Zap the Attitude. How tragic it is that anyone, let alone many of us, do not respect ourselves or prize ourselves as being worthy, or of having value. I have felt a certain sense of horror when I realised this about myself, it is very sad and quite huge developmentally and from a self-care point of view. I sit here with an outpouring of love for anyone (and myself) who have found themselves in that situation depleted of their own self-worth, disregarding and dismissing themselves of their own needs, because they don't matter.

If this is true for you too, I invite you to sit with that feeling whilst giving yourself a big dollop of self-compassion. You 'owe' it to yourself to give yourself that time and attention.

It is a process like any other, that we need to learn to do differently, in order to learn how to meet our own needs. We all have needs, just like a car does, just like a phone needs to be plugged in to recharge as I keep saying! Learning how to value ourselves, respect ourselves, treat ourselves with dignity and regard to allow ourselves to know that we do matter.

## 3. Valuing Ourselves

Valuing ourselves is a big concept in self-care and can be very difficult to do! I'm generalising, but I wonder if it is up there as one of the most difficult, 'unnatural' things for therapists who are 'prone' to over-giving, to learn to do. Paying attention to ourselves means that we value ourselves. Acknowledging and accepting as a given that we have needs much like accepting the petrol needs of the car, to fuel it. The attention, that we pay, to ourselves is an energy investment. I'll repeat that because in energetic terms it's important. The attention, that we pay, to ourselves is an energy investment. Energy follows attention. Attention and that focus on ourselves sends a message back to us that we are worth it, that we deserve it and that we matter.

If we don't value ourselves, how can we expect others to? The process often starts with us taking action first on that front. It isn't an automatic thing that we can demand that others appreciate and value us first, often it can be that the responsibility starts with us. If we are lucky we may have a nice nudge from a kind person who treats us well, that reminds us of those around us who don't - as well as ourselves. Those who have experienced abuse on any level, may still be carrying the old wounds and scars of that trauma which leads them to find that they experience repeated situations where they aren't valued or considered (and worse). Energy Clearing (see the Energy Hygiene section) may help clear some of that and possibly the shamanic practise of soul retrieval to help recover parts of the soul that might have left due to shock or trauma. I noticed significant benefit from the practise of soul retrieval myself and noticed a gradual strengthening in what I felt able to do, with firmer boundaries and a sense of being more intact.

## So what are you worth?

In learning about valuing ourselves, I remember a story that a therapist told about someone phoning her up to ask how much she charged for her sessions. This has always stayed with me in terms of remembering my value. She stated her price clearly to the person who was enquiring about the amount that she charged (which was a reasonable, fairly average rate). They said 'Great, I'll go with you, you obviously know your worth'. Having faith in ourselves and the skills that we have and what we can offer as a service for them, can also transmit a message of confidence to the other person, that we can deliver on some level or other. Knowing our value, can really help to convey that.

We may also like to consider if are we deserving of receiving something for our time? There may be, as mentioned previously, the belief that the spiritual life is one of poverty – the concept of non-attachment to material possessions is indicative of how much we are able to let go and trust that we will be provided for and isn't the path for everyone.

Feeling uncomfortable about accepting money can be a theme which also shows itself in the same vein as feeling uncomfortable about receiving (and believing) compliments – the discomfort can highlight that on some level we do not feel worthy to receive. If we can learn to give to ourselves by realistically acknowledging our own needs, by that act we are honouring and acknowledging our worth, and valuing ourselves. It can be a slow process but we then begin to see that we too are worthy to receive. If we fulfil our own needs, ultimately by doing so we can give more to others if and when we decide in some circumstances that we do want to give freely.

## 3. Valuing Ourselves

In Reiki, it is said that Usui, the founder of Reiki, found that the treatments were working initially, but they were not holding long-term for people and they became ill again. He found that when he introduced a charge for treatments, that this seemed to work better. By paying for a treatment people can participate more fully in their own recovery, by the process of taking responsibility for their health. I certainly found this to be the case from my own journey to wellbeing. I look back and see how much I have flourished and grown and how they have also helped me to do my job that I love.

Some people do prefer to pay; it can be a matter of pride that they do not want to feel indebted to another if they themselves are not used to receiving something for nothing, 'unconditionally'. If we refuse to take something that someone is offering, we may offend them, by saying no. If we like to give, surely we can then see that another likes to give also. If we consider this in energetic terms, when we say 'no', we are blocking the flow of energy, putting up resistance and barriers and one of the keys is to keep positive energy flowing constantly otherwise it backs up and becomes blocked. By staying open and saying yes, we thus keep the flow of energy (in this example money) going.

It is interesting also to consider that the man who enquired about the price of the therapist seemed to be of the opinion that if there is not a sufficient price on something, then it holds less of a value. Some lack belief in a treatment working or being any good if a fair price isn't charged (others if an extortionate one isn't charged but I would draw the line at that personally and morally!). They may be of the belief that 'we get what we pay for' and the more that they pay, the more they will get. Above a certain price I'm not sure that this is quite true of therapies!

I have treatments weekly, for my own health and well-being and I also benefit from them in a CPD way. The therapist may help me in some way that can then go on to benefit my clients, whether that's highlighting something about my own practise and way of working or a technique or an aspect of anatomy and physiology that I learn from what they are doing for me. Also if I am giving to so many clients weekly it's a good part of energy hygiene, i.e. it helps to clear my energy. Paying for those treatments sends me a strong self- care message that I am worth it, that I am of value.

There have been times when my finances have been stretched and I've felt like I've needed to try to cut corners and have longer periods between treatments or less time, etc. However, I always feel that pinch on a personal energy level, because I don't feel so good about myself and things don't then tend to flow in my life. Bookings may drop off - which then start up again when I engage in my commitment to self-care. I liken it to plugging in.

## Manifesting or co-creating

Trusting that the money will be there to pay for my well-being is a large part of valuing and trusting my connection with the flow of life and it's abundance. If I 'keep showing up' (ie participating in the process of the flow of life) and doing my best for others (in service to the Divine and passing that flow of energy on), I am taken care of and the finances will be there for me to do that. This is a process, sometimes called Manifesting or Co-Creating, which doesn't happen overnight, but like much of this, is a journey that over time we can come to navigate and trust. I won't go into it here, but trying something like the 21 days abundance meditation practise that Deepak Chopra set up online for others to share or reading some of the books that are out there on this subject can help you to understand that process further. During the lead up to my first stint at writing this book I had two treatments that week, and whilst writing it, another to keep my inspirational energy levels high and the ideas flowing - the money was there for me to do that, as it was for me to go away. I truly value and am grateful for that source of abundance in my life and now over time my trust that I am cared for by God and the Universal Resources, as I show up and do my bit, is reinforced time and time again. It is a beautiful process, but hasn't always been that way!

## Cancellation charges

As well as charging for our services, valuing ourselves enough to charge for cancellations was another big step where I felt I had to stick my neck out. I went through a period of time and then especially over one week where I had so many cancellations that I realised that I couldn't afford to not put a boundary in place, on that level, at that time. Whilst I appreciate many cancellations were genuine, as I myself have made errors with turning up for my own appointments from time to time, I also intuited that there were some who were not valuing and considering me as a person who needs to pay their bills too. I needed to protect myself and my energy levels as it was depleting me. At that time some clients were just not showing up without telling me and others were just forgetting and I wondered why this was happening in my life, what it was showing me and what I could do to rectify it.

I saw that a number of others therapists and institutions had begun to charge for cancellations or no shows. I reasoned that if I lost clients who weren't going to respect the time that I had put aside for them and their appointment, then so be it. At least my energy levels would be protected and in that way I took care of myself. I put up a notice in my room to inform clients that if there were cancellations within the 24 hours they would be charged. It can take considerable time and effort to reappoint clients, with texts going backwards and forwards (the preferred mode of contact nowadays).

I now also have an online booking system which should help with a lot of that. The majority of clients were very understanding about the cancellation policy and most are willing to pay, as I too always offer myself if I've made an error and forgotten an appointment with someone myself. They have a business to run, as do I.

If I can slot someone else in, then I won't charge the person who has cancelled, because I don't want to charge someone for something that I haven't done, however I do also need to be clear that it is wasteful of my time if someone isn't genuinely wanting to engage in treatments. I find that it just makes people think a bit more before booking. Interestingly, now that my levels of trust have deepened further, I am noticing again (as I had initially) that those times where someone doesn't show up can be filled in other ways that my Universal diary planner has more of an idea about than I do. In that I mean that it may give me that time to do other things such as admin or clean my room. I am now at a point where I am going to experiment with a new notice where a mention of repeated cancellations may incur a cancellation fee.

## Freebies and exchanges

Over the years of working with clients holistically I have provided free treatments and been involved in not for profit organisations, I've done exchanges with other therapists, I've allowed donations and sometimes they do work out. By that I mean that some clients really do value them, and I am not taken for a ride, or I haven't put myself out at the EXPENSE of another. Giving to others can be draining and not everyone appreciates that energy as we might appreciate it ourselves. I tune in to my intuition and ask how to proceed when considering a scenario of exchange or donation and I still don't always get it right but then that does teach me!

Time has a value and when we do exchanges with another it may not always work out equally; money can simplify things in many ways. To say I've done a treatment for someone and given an hour of my time with the expenditure of effort may not be equal to the expenditure of effort it has take someone to do something else for an hour, it maybe more or less. On that note I think domestic/cleaning staff should be paid much more than they are as they are cleaning up after other people's stuff! What a job! Much kudos to them caring for us in that way. Maybe if we could turn our system of valuing around, the world may turn on its head too!

My understanding of valuing myself deepened when I was offering discount to a client and I had problems with my roof, which my mum was paying for. I'd not long started working again and couldn't afford it. The client to who I was giving discount said they were paying for windows to be done on their house. It might have been his mother paying for it too, but it did hit me like a ton of roofing slate that I did need to value myself more as I needed really to be paying for my own roof! (and look at how symbolic that was too). It was and is about priorities sometimes too - how much does someone value their own health or their windows? Sometimes it can be as simple (or complicated) a choice as that.

# I'm not worth it

Over the years I have noticed that clients that come for treatments which are free or on offer are often not likely to be the ones that (can/want to or do) pay full price. People's limitations in terms of valuing their own health and what they are worth, and what they are prepared to pay is something that many seem to battle with. Sometimes that might be because they aren't in great need, or don't feel like they are a priority; it can sometimes feel like that when there are other bills to pay. At base level it can also be that we aren't fully valuing ourselves in some way. I've noticed that therapists and givers may often be either reluctant to engage in paid treatments or promise themselves that they will do it more often but then don't! Is this true for you?

# Valuing our time

As I mentioned in over-giving, sometimes we can give our time away to others all too easily. I explained the scenario where I was giving too much time at work because I didn't feel like an hour was 'enough'. The friend who just phones up when they want to moan, because you have a good listening ear or the one that drops round for a coffee because they are bored and you are often available, can 'take' time. If we get something out of this too, it may be fine, but if we start to feel tired or depleted it could be that we are spending too much time on others and perhaps not valuing our own time.

Characteristic of a highly sensitive person is the need to have time alone. When we appreciate that this is what we have to do to recharge, we often come to value that time and that space to replenish. A common criticism of those who are not willing to pay for energy therapies is that if it is spiritual it should be free. For those with the expectation that Reiki or any healing should be free of charge, it may be worth considering how much they value healing and how much they value their health. If they are unwell, do you see them taking responsibility for their own health and doing what they can to return to health - not necessarily what we think they should be doing but making their own efforts? How do you yourself feel about paying for treatments? It could be that your experiences with others are reflecting back something about yourself.

When I encountered individuals who felt that it was their right to have something for nothing, a sense of entitlement, it eventually gave me more backbone to realise that I needed to value myself, when others didn't. It does need to start with ourselves. When we value ourselves and know our self-worth, other people take note.

And the come back from therapists to 'spiritual healing should be free' has often been 'you are not paying for the energy but you are paying for my time'. When we work with more and more people and don't have another job to pay the bills, it might be a decision that we make to value our time and put a price on that in order to replenish ourselves so that we can be of more consistent benefit to others.

## Donations and trust

Another consideration is to work with a system of donations if we find it difficult to put a price on our services or even want to use this system as a great surrender to trust in the universe. However, many people in my experience do not know how to respond to a donation system. They wonder what to pay, wondering what the going rate is. A 'suggested donation' maybe on a sliding scale of £15 - £80 for instance, which can give people a loose guideline. Using a system of donation we are also placing our trust in the Universe that we will be provided for, and letting go of the outcome and expectation.

The process of donating is one of handing responsibility of what something is worth to the person that is receiving. This enables the recipient to consider what they can really afford and how much they truly value what they are receiving, whilst acknowledging and taking into account differing circumstances.

## Depleting Activities

On the opposite end of the spectrum to valuing ourselves, where we are cherishing and nurturing ourselves, are those things that we do which can deplete us. Often known as depleting activities, it can help us to be aware of these so that we can understand how better to value or take care of ourselves and the ways that we can do this. Noticing or finding things that deplete us and making adjustment can stop us from leaking energy. I personally find that if I take my phone up to the bedroom, I don't like the feel of the energy plus it's too stimulating for me as well as too tempting to suddenly google something I've been thinking about. It makes for a more restful wind down and sleep for me if I don't have it, so as part of valuing myself and regarding that, I self-ban it.

Being with people that we don't like can be particularly depleting, it might be that those people are critical, judgemental, controlling, narcissistic or something else you just can't put your finger on so you may be better off limiting your time with them, sometimes even cutting off your relationship with someone may be necessary if you have tried unsuccessfully to reach a compromise. I love the phrase 'those that matter don't mind and those that mind don't matter'.

Another epiphany that I had was that I didn't have to be liked by everyone. This may seem obvious to some, but when self-worth is low it may be determined by whether we are accepted by others or not, being social creatures it is a fundamental survival strategy. I then realised I had a choice. I understood that because I didn't particularly like some people, realistically not everyone was going to like me either, and I could 'reject' people (i.e. I had a choice to accept them in my life or not, I don't mean that in an unkindly way). It was a relief. Life can be made much harder by trying too hard to get on with people who just simply aren't on the same wavelength, or we just don't feel the same about.

Christmas time especially can be a difficult time for many people and can become a depleting activity, when in many ways it 'should' be about value and cherishing, yet brings up all sorts of issues such as materialism and stress. Break the cycle of whatever it is at Christmas (if you 'celebrate' or even chose not to), rectifying if you can that which unsettles or upsets you. Spend time with those you feel truly comfortable with, be true to yourself. I particularly love this time of year now to ask for inspiration for the giving of gifts. I ask for ideas that will bring happiness and pleasure to others and feel a real joy in trusting that the finances will be there to benefit those that I give to.

## Someone's depletion may be another's gain

I struggled for years (to the point of meltdowns) to do my accounts for work. No matter how hard I concentrate I literally can make 2 + 2 add up to 5. Fortunately I had some support, account wise, from family, but I made the decision to hand it over completely to be done by an accountant, because I knew realistically no matter how hard I tried I would make mistakes. I had to accept that it was depleting me and stressed me considerably and I ask the universe for the treatments to come in so that I can pay someone else to do what they are good at - this is what makes the world go round. I don't have to carry it all on my shoulders! And nor do you.

I love this philosophy, because when we are doing what we enjoy and what we are good at, we can then pay - and value - someone else to do the work which puts food on their table too. Holding onto money stops the flow of abundance. When we 'fear' we don't have enough money it blocks the flow, if we takes steps towards trust, we can release it. What can you hand over to someone else to do?

One of my more difficult delegations is that of allowing clients to book in online. Doing my job and booking people in is quite time consuming, as I can't answer the phone whilst doing treatments. I have had a few therapists do this and it felt very unboundaried, as if someone else was in the room! Texts can go back and forth, especially if there is a bit of chatter going on between myself and clients. This can sometimes be in the evening when I get round to doing it if I don't have time in between treatments, which means I'm working later. I have really come to value my time at home now as rest time and whilst sometimes it's ok, and quite nice, to answer texts in the evening, I don't always have the energy. Having an online booking system is something that I have to let go of my own worries and concerns about and go with, because it will save me a considerable amount of time and energy. Change can be hard but we can adjust. As it is just being trialled, it is lovely to get a text message pop up that just says that a booking has been made without the back and forth that can sometimes happen and frees me up a little.

## Slow suicide

I'll conclude this chapter with some real food for thought and maybe even a bit of a wake-up call. Bluntly put, how many of us engage in slow suicide in one form or other? If we look in black and white terms about the degree of care that we take for ourselves, how we treat ourselves, how we nurture ourselves and how we deplete or even harm ourselves, are we truly valuing our lives?

Having lived for many years when I could put no value on my own life and I literally had a death wish, I had no gratitude or appreciation for my life because it felt so frequently raw, painful and nonsensical. It has been a long slow journey to find those missing elements that have anchored me in a reality where contentment, acceptance, peace and joy are more common feelings for me. Yet there is still growth and work to be done. Consequently I, like many others in life, knowingly make what I would prefer to think of as 'unskilled choices'. Were I to be completely mindful and upholding of my well-being, those choices would be different. I would eat far less refined sugar, I would rise at 5am and rest at 9pm, I would do this that and the other. But I'm as human as you too are, reading this. Judging ourselves for what we do or don't do will not likely help, but discerning how we can make more skilled choices may. My point is that in black and white terms I know those choices are still ones that don't fine tune or benefit me. They are as they are for now, I am open to changing them and doing differently and welcome looking at ways to do that.

# 3. Valuing Ourselves

How many of us can, in all honesty, acknowledge that what we are doing to ourselves is detrimental in the long-term? We may not have a direct intention of killing ourselves, but over time is the choice to smoke not a slow-suicide? Is binge drinking and its impact on the liver 'wearing' you out? Is lack of five a day like running your car on empty? And is going for a run whilst not paying attention to your emotional health and grievances running yourself into the ground? Can we admit to ourselves that perhaps our view of self-care is not as we would perhaps advise our clients? Can we humbly admit to ourselves that we would benefit from learning to walk our talk better? What dissatisfactions are these 'coping mechanisms' covering up in our lives and how can we fill those gaps or mend them in ways that are healthy? How can we learn to value ourselves better?

Understanding what our true value is, is a journey of discovering who we really are, what our values are and what we value in life too. Do we value our own life? It might be a combination of valuing who we are and what we do. Do we value certain qualities in others such as genuineness and authenticity, and kindness or do we revel in what they actually do? And what qualities do we then value in ourselves? And what other things do we value about ourselves? What traits or achievements come to mind about you? What skills do you have? How are you unique as a being? How can you truly come to value yourself better to mend that gap?

# Chapter Four

## Prioritising Your Time

Prioritising may be obvious to some people, it might come naturally.

It might, however, be something that those of us with self care blocks may struggle with. The definition of prioritising in the Oxford English dictionary is to 'designate or treat (something) as being very or most important and 'determine the order for dealing with (a series of items or tasks) according to their relative importance'

We may habitually and automatically put our own needs way down the list sending ourselves a message that we aren't important. Our internal programming might be that the end goal of pleasing someone and making everyone else happy is a priority. It is often that we can be making those survival choices from childhood, (or adulthood if we have experienced long term abusive relationships). We may have the thought if we live with someone difficult, 'anything for an easy life', where we just roll over and conform, even if that is at a long term cost to us.

## I don't matter

However, when we keep putting ourselves aside for others, putting their needs higher up the list than ours, we send a message to ourselves, albeit unconsciously, that we don't matter,  we aren't important and that we don't value ourselves. It might be that on some level we believe that other people are more important than us, that we aren't a priority - and sometimes we aren't. However, to not even notice our own wants and needs can cause them to become suppressed.

As a consequence of not having even been conscious of my needs for years, I began a process of tuning myself 'back into me' which brings me back to myself. I ask myself on waking: 'What do I want to do today?', I tune in and notice how I feel. I pay attention to me. Paying attention to ourselves is an 'energy' investment, we are 'giving' ourselves energy. I then assess whether my wants and needs are realistic, or not, or how I can try to accommodate others if there are conflicting priorities. I also set an intention when this is the case, that I be guided for the greater good of all. That might not necessarily be what I think is for the best at the time, but if I take that advice or intuition, it can unfold that it does work out to be for the best.

Coming away to Aberystwyth to write again, my goal was to make real headway on the first draft, so that the content was mainly there and finished. On the way there I noticed a cold coming on. I got on quite well the following day despite feeling a bit rough. Checking in with what felt best for me I decided against going for a run. I often still go if it's only mild as it can help, but that day I walked instead. On waking the next morning, I felt lousy. I was also ravenous. Feed a cold. So although my plan generally was to either go out for a run first thing then write, and have something to eat later I decided again no run, but walk for breakfast.

## Internal arguments

My inner Sergeant Major (my ego) was having a bit of a rant at this, 'not going to get this finished, blah blah', whilst my soul says 'trust; you know how things unfold'. I was experiencing the conflict of what were my priorities and my focus, with not feeling well. I had to adapt and be more flexible from my original plans. This also meant that I had a good example to illustrate. So my needs to take care of myself, by having a protein rich breakfast which would set me up for the day sent a message to myself that I matter. The book does too, but also trusting that something greater than the Sergeant Major (The Powers that Be, who I thank for trying to take care of me) has the big picture or plan in mind.

My first awareness of this 'priorities' business, wasn't until my early twenties. During a better spell of health, I'd invited some friends round for a barbecue for my birthday. I started cleaning the house in a frenzy and began to get quite stressed about what I wanted to get done, as well as preparing some of the food. My sister quite rightly pointed out that my friends were coming to see me, not my house and explained a bit about priorities, just to get done what I could. I'd never thought of life in that way before. I was thinking in terms of Sergeant Major mode, of 'what I had to get done'. This is about the inner thoughts and pressure that I put myself under. I'd absorbed the unrealistic expectations of others around me and that had become my inner programming or driver. This can be societies expectations, parents, guardians way of doing things that until we question whether they are right for us just drive us subconsciously. Instead I could reframe it as 'what I want to get done'. There can be a difference between what we want to do and what's ideal for us, and what we need to do and also what we realistically can do?

Are we over pressuring ourselves in Sergeant Major mode? Can we thank our inner Sergeant Major's for organising us and helping us to get things done on other occasions? We can say to ourselves that instead, the approach of our 'helpful compassion' is more suited to working with us today, on this one. Thereby we get done what we realistically can, rather than what we 'should' do?

## Dependent others

I'd like to point out the obvious, that there is a difference with parenting. Children's needs are frequently a priority and parents are responsible for their children's safety and care. By the very nature of child rearing, those children's needs often do come before their own, such as getting up to feed them at night and sacrificing sleep. However, that fine balance of the pilot on the plane saying to parents 'put your own oxygen mask on first' is important. How can you save your child if you aren't alive to do it? Also, as children get older, their needs may lessen as a priority as they grow. Their skill development and learning may benefit from doing things themselves - see the butterfly story in Healer Heal Thyself.

The other challenging scenario is a dependent other that we may be caring for, such as an immobile parent. There maybe respite services and carer support organisations that you can investigate, which can help to take a small amount of pressure off. Having worked with carers via a variety of local organisations, I see how difficult and challenging that role really is and my heart goes out to anyone in that situation. Not for one instance am I saying it's easy, nor that what I am saying is the right way to go. We all have to find what's right within ourselves and our own way through. But our priorities should never mean that someone else is in danger. Unfortunately, that can be the real crux of the choice, when carers feel trapped by circumstance, and a lack of support. It's because of this that local organisations in my area do have schemes where they will send the carers for holistic therapy treatments in efforts to boost them up. And it's always worth remembering - do you allow yourself to be supported?

## Prioritising others needs

Another example that springs to mind about prioritising others needs is when my ex-partner decided to transition from male to female. He had not long been made redundant from work whilst in hospital with cellulitis and we were on holiday in Cornwall. We were sitting in the car outside the holiday cottage, just talking and he said to me that he felt that he wanted to cross dress more. He was nervous about it because he wasn't sure where it would take him and what it would open up, and his fear was that we would break up.

Not long after we first met, he told me that he was transgender. This was something that in the past I often thought I wouldn't be able to accept, because of magazine articles with ramped up drama about how wives were shocked to come home and discover their husbands in women's underwear. However, here was someone who was being honest and open, and although I felt nervous about going into the unknown, I had mentally explored the concept of lesbian relationships, so wasn't closed to that. Over the years though he rarely presented as a female. When he did, it took some moments to adjust to - just like someone with a new hair cut.

Here we were in Cornwall, sat in the car. I was scared. Would we get bricks through the window as I'd feared when he first told me about this. Would he be misunderstood? I tuned into my soul and my feelings. Very clearly I felt that I would need to put myself aside, but it felt very right to support my partner in this. I said to him that I couldn't honestly say how I would feel should he transition, rather than just (cross dress) every now and then, because I'd not been in that position before. The great thing was that we had always been able to be very open and honest with each other.

The long and short of it was that we went off for the first shopping trip of many, and after we were home from holiday it was only a short while that he transitioned and began to live full time as a female. This did need an adjustment as I had to get used to her new name, and also the time she took in the bathroom now! We told our families and then friends and they were extremely supportive. I realised that this intense transformation process would take a lot of energy, the person is changing so much in many ways including the way that they relate to you and you to them. There is a grieving process as you are losing the person that was and also the part of you that related to the person that they were, that part dies within you. Even though in many ways they are essentially the same 'essence' of the person that was, in many ways there are also big differences. We joked that he was buried under the patio! So there was sadness.

I consciously put myself aside on numerous occasions during this process, however, it was mindful and I also took the best care that I could of myself during that time. I knew that self care was paramount; that the process of transformation is understandably self-absorbed and I also had my own emotional and mental needs too. However, it then got to a point where I was depleted, despite my conscious self-care plan and my needs weren't being met in the relationship. I experienced a pivotal moment during an exercise in a counselling class where we were asked to draw a crystal, then describe it. Extremely Freudian in my response, I realised that my needs as well as part of my identity were about me being in a heterosexual relationship. Complicated by or spurred on by this, I had met someone else through a group. I felt a strong pull and I didn't want to have an affair and although the timing didn't seem great, life was pointing me in another direction, I was now becoming a priority again.

Relationship break ups are often the crux of a priority process where we begin to assess our needs and whether they are being met, and start to pay attention to ourselves as we become more of a priority. It was also part of a soul decision for me, which also reflected aspects of the wounded healer. It was distressing to see how much pain my ex-partner was feeling from the break up and in that I had to distance myself to quite a degree. My mum had said at the time of transition, 'no matter what happens, you'll always be best friends'. My soul very much said that this was the right thing to do and that she would grow and her life would be better as a consequence of our split. She would have to spread her wings like the butterfly and that one day she'd understand this too.

I love the saying  'And the day came when the risk to remain tight in a bud was more painful than the risk it took to blossom' by Anais Nin, because life can be hard and painful temporarily. Undoubtedly our time together helped us both to grow into the people that we are today and as a result we are doing well on our separate paths. We are both now in very happy relationships and are still the best of friends.

# Questions to ask ourselves when prioritising

It can be difficult and confusing, trying to prioritise our needs. As I mentioned previously, on waking I tune into myself to see how I feel physically and mentally. 'What do I want?' is a question you can ask yourself to get a sense of where you are at within yourself. If you don't know where you are at, you can't honestly relate to others. This is where our 'don't know' answers can come in and we may end up committing to doing something we don't really want to do, or don't feel able to do and then feeling resentful about that or cancelling.

Despite having done this for many years I still forget sometimes too; it is a process of learning to remember sometimes as we can find ourselves in situations which trigger us to 'forget ourselves'. After checking in with myself, I then ask myself 'Do I want to go for a run?' if I have one 'planned' (loosely), will it benefit me? What's going on today, what are my energy levels like, etc.? Throughout the day I check-in with myself on this basis, knowing that there has to be a degree of flexibility and that things can change. I have had to learn to do this, because I didn't have a strong sense of myself at all, so would frequently end up saying I'd do things without really wanting to, which then often led to me letting people down. I didn't have a strong sense of myself and possibly, like yourself, I wasn't a priority.

The following questions may help you to sort through some confusion that you may have about prioritising. These can also be done alongside the practise that is in the Answers are Within, which is in part II of the book. For now, just take a breath, meditate, relax and maybe get your journal out if you have one or make a note on some paper, maybe even recording the questions and pausing to give you time to reflect may help you to focus. Ask yourself any of the following that might be relevant to your situation:

- What is my need in this moment? Do I need more time? What needs to be done? What doesn't need to be done?

- What is their need in this moment? (Separate the two, people who are enmeshed - see the Boundaries section - might not know the difference and think that the others need and their own need is the same)

- Realistically what may happen if I don't do this, what are the consequences? How might I feel (note, might, rather than how will I feel - in reality we may not feel like we anticipate)

## 'Priority time' for you!

Do you give yourself any time? I don't mean time to go swimming or time out with friends. I mean gaps in your diary where you aren't rushing from A to B. Often we may fill our days and our diaries and be so busy that we don't even have space to breathe, going from one thing to another. I am just washing the t-shirt for this one myself, so I have taken it off, but I'm working on it!

Giving ourselves time gives us space, which is important so we don't overload ourselves. Can you give yourself time. And if not, what do you fear by creating that space or that void? What is it about that emptiness? What would emerge if we did give ourselves that time? What are we avoiding or preventing by not giving ourselves time?

As with all of the self-care obstacles there are fundamental reasons why we don't do things or why we do do things. Until we are ready to look at them and let them go, it can help just to observe what we are doing and just say to ourselves 'there's me again, leaving myself no time'. That may also be a timing thing in itself, when the right time comes and we are ready and have sufficient tools in our self-care tool kit, we may then look at why we aren't giving ourselves that time. But for now, just notice. I sat and tuned in to this aspect myself and achievement is a big thing for me. My inner Sergeant Major can sometimes aggressively say 'must do better, must do more', instead of my spirit which kindly says 'enough's enough and that is good enough'.

## The building of Rome

Another facet of giving ourselves time is the unrealistic expectation that we will understand and put into practise the things that we have learnt in a self-help book straight away. Some people may pick up aspects of it very quickly and make rapid and significant changes straight away, but for the majority of us it can take years chipping away at the old programmes. Hypnotherapy, Energy Therapy and shamanic soul retrieval work, may help some in speeding up that process, but realistically, acknowledging that we are a lifelong process can help us to take the pressure off achieving things here and now. Knowing that life is a journey can help quieten that inner critical voice that many of us have, which says 'you've failed'.

I tend to think of it all as a learning experience; life teaches me. If something isn't working or I'm taking my time to learn it, I often find it's because there is more for me to learn about myself or about the processes or techniques for my inner 'toolkit'.

## Right timing

I like the saying 'There is a time for everything and a season for every activity'. It is so true that when the time is right, things do just unfold and flow naturally. Life becomes much easier. Until then we may be inclined to force things, wrestle with ourselves and overstretch ourselves because the time just isn't right. This is not an attitude of compassionate self-care; this is coming from the ego.

Sometimes we may benefit from backing right off of ourselves and supporting ourselves rather than trying to flog ourselves to death! With that sort of mentality, brute force and lack of self-empathy to get things done, it seems arrogant and a form of superiority that we are greater than the Powers that Be, God or the Universal Flow.

## We don't always get to the traffic lights when they are on green

I appreciate phrases that come through in readings, as they teach me too. I'm always mindful of this, and I particularly like this phrase. So things aren't happening, they aren't going to plan, they're not unfolding as we would want them to. One of the phrases that has helped me to understand that it's OK to have these times in life, and comes through repeatedly during readings for people and makes so much sense is that 'we don't always get to the traffic lights when they are on green'. It might be that we sit there impatiently at the lights, even cursing, but most of us generally accept that we will wait our turn and the red light means 'don't go yet'. It could be dangerous if we do and traffic lights are there to keep us safe ultimately - not to hold us up. However knowing that our ego, ever the controller, is trying to tell us that we are the be all and end all of the universe and that the lights, or timing generally SHOULD be changing, just doesn't work. We know that eventually if everything is in order the lights do go to green.

The same is true of the flow of life and juggling those priorities and our time. We often stress about things that we really have no control over anyway. I love the Serenity prayer *'Grant me the serenity to accept the things that I cannot change, courage to change the things I can and the wisdom to know the difference'*. This can help to relinquish some of those feelings of control that we may be holding onto and as we let go, it can give us that important time and space to relax. Sending some of our experiences up to the Divine or out to the Universe can help life to flow, so that ultimately we all benefit.

# Chapter Five

## Owning our Shadow

### Shadow work

The truly free spirit can allow themselves to be tethered, and surrender gracefully because their reality knows there really are no binds, the self proclaimed free spirit on the other hand may fear attachment and responsibility, and merely be running scared.

As part of our self-care plan, it can help us to become aware of our shadow selves. These are the parts that we bury away and push down inside us, preferring not to recognise within ourselves, such as anger and jealousy for example. Our 'shadow' aspects are those things that we might not want to deal with, sometimes because it is too painful to look at. The aspects are buried, out of our awareness, our 'blind spot' and in the realms of the unconscious until, for example, moments of stress, where they may leak out and we may have experiences where our feelings are out of our control. Our shadow selves are often aspects that those close to us are aware of and see within us anyway, we just don't recognise it within ourselves. A good example of this is the angry peace protester. The anger is repressed and the person demands peace, but internally isn't peaceful and when cornered the anger spills out.

We can overreact when a repressed issue triggers or fuels our behaviour in the present moment. It can be the unconscious repressed parts of ourselves that are surfacing or emerging 'into the light', in order to be addressed and resolved. This can come after the breakdown of the persona, i.e. a breakdown or a period where we can feel 'shattered' or in pieces.

For example, our partner triggers an overreaction in us and we 'explode'. We may wonder why we feel as strongly as we do, and have awareness that we might be 'over the top'. We may come to realise that we have suppressed our anger and are very angry ourselves towards someone else about something in the past and we project (or dump) it onto our partner in the present.

When parts of us are in shadow, or repressed, we may numb or deaden ourselves when we split off the emotions. Activities such as over-eating, drinking, drugs, extreme sports or over-giving which may then help us to feel 'alive' again or keep the emotions that may threaten to overwhelm us at bay.

Within relationships, if partners do not take ownership and responsibility for their issues, we can continue to blame each other. Relationships may be shallow and superficial, lacking depth and arguments may escalate and feel out of control. Problems are unresolved, if partners see themselves in only a positive light and the other as the one at fault, rather than understanding that there is good and bad in all of us.

## Extra self-care

The shadow is the term for 'everything that we can't see within ourselves', so by its nature it can often be a shock to realise something about ourselves that we weren't aware of. For this reason, and because it can be painful, working with our shadow necessitates a large degree of self-compassion. This means having an ability to listen to ourselves, without judging ourselves, but accepting that we are as we are.

The process of working with the shadow can cause upheaval in our lives due to changes in our perception, we start to see things differently which can open us up. We may view other people in our lives very differently.

Other self-care practises to support us in shadow work are learning how to ground, which is covered in the energy hygiene section, making sure that we get out in nature, and taking exercise, as well as eating a wholesome diet to support us in this journey. Mindfulness techniques can be very effective at allowing us to sit with and breathe into feelings. Noticing with non-judgemental awareness these characteristics can then allow us to own them. Just noticing the feelings that we have, such as greed, and accepting that 'they are as they are' helps us to calm our overreactions to these so called negative aspects of ourselves. By not judging them but knowing that each of us is really doing the best that we can, that they are often coping or defence mechanisms that have tried to keep us safe in someway, we can be grateful that they have served a purpose.

Having a good network of supportive people that you can rely on and letting them know that you are doing personal development work and shadow work and might be challenged may be a good idea. If there are deeper issues that have caused you problems, it may be an idea to skip this chapter (or proceed with caution) and seek the help of someone who is trained in this area. Journaling as an outlet to let it all out is another helpful way, or finding a Jungian or transpersonal therapist, a spiritual life coach, a shamanic practitioner or therapist who embraces shadow work and what it entails.

Energy therapies and energy hygiene can also help, e.g. meditation, clearing work, Reiki, Angel Therapy, Diamond Energy Therapy, etc., just to keep heavy energy shifting and clearing.

The father of shadow work was the psychologist Carl Jung. Other resources and authors who deal with it are Debbie Ford, John Monbourquette and Caroline Myss. Shadow work does come with a warning, but it can also be transformational and liberating.

## A psychic virus

During a hypnosis session many years ago, I recalled an event from the past and saw the person throwing toxic black energy towards and onto me as I took that in. I saw others having done the same to him and a process where everyone passes this from one person to the next, if they don't deal with it or take responsibility for their 'stuff'. It's like a psychic, energetic, virus.

This is talked about in People of the Lie by M Scott Peck and in Dispelling Wetiko by Paul Levy. Wetiko is a name for the dark energy that I had seen passed to me which can be passed from one person to another, down ancestral lines, and feeds the shadow part of us. It is in us all to one degree or another, it is just like psychic pollution. When we shine a light on this darkness, and notice it (but not pay too much attention to it, not to feed it!) it help us to stop the cycle. Owning those parts of us that can be grumpy, rude, irritable, lazy or angry can help to prevent this toxic shadow side of us from controlling us, so we don't act it out and dump it on another. When we can accept without judging ourselves, 'I can be a bit mean and selfish', breathe into it and just be aware, the shadow loses its momentum and grip.

## Why do shadow work?

Shadow work can lead us to emotional maturity, responding from an integrated perspective rather than a 'split' off or repressed childish part. We begin to cultivate more awareness and become more conscious of our behaviour as well as our feelings. Shadow work can help the parts of us that battle internally between 'right and wrong' or 'this and that' to quieten.

By taking responsibility for our own shadow we may notice that our relationships are strengthened, because we are less likely to project those shadow aspects onto friends and partners. We become less reactive and emotionally charged with others, and as we become more compassionate of ourselves and our own faults, we can also be more forgiving of others and their faults too. Our consciousness also becomes wider and stronger.

Personal honesty is about noticing our true feelings and emotions and accepting them as they are without judgement. It can be hard to look at our agendas and motives, realising that we may have manipulative behaviours that drive us. Noticing these with discernment can lead us to accept our humanness and promote integrity.

Shadow work also opens up our illusions, we are not so likely to be naively taken in, as we begin to recognise the shadow in others too, for what it is. The perspective of accepting that 'we are all trying to get our needs met' and there are various ways of doing that, conscious and unconscious, can be quite grounding.

## Running from the shadows

I've often thought about the runners, or the person who is supposedly super fit, who suddenly die of heart failure and everyone is shocked. However, holistically when we push down our emotions into the shadow, it may have a physical affect on the body. I suspect this is quite often the case with fibromyalgia, ME, IBS and possibly other illnesses. So it might be that the runner, who has put their all into their running, is focusing on their physical fitness, but running away from their emotional 'fitness', possibly old heartache. Only that person themselves would be able to comment on that; I'm not a believer in one size fits all, but it does fit some. Certainly I noticed that for me, running helped to work out the old 'fight or flight' energy, whilst I worked on the mental and emotional issues too. Now I feel less of a flight energy to run, to work that energy out, as it isn't such an issue and I enjoy a more mindful run.

Within spiritual communities it can be seen as ideal to be 'pure' and live in 'love and light'. However, maintenance of this 'persona', can cause fear, anger, sadness, jealousy and other shadow aspects to be repressed, which can then lead to scapegoating, and blaming behaviours. This then leaves people feeling insufficient, guilty and shameful for not being able to reach these high ideals, which can lead to a feeling of the person being unreal or inauthentic and incongruent.

Sometimes called 'spiritual bypassing', when we don't take ownership of our shadow qualities, and instead give an impression or have a persona of 'the good guy', our shadow traits can leak out particularly during times of stress, causing us to over react or blame others, for faults or issues that are really ours.

In short, our shadow can be how we are with those who are closest to us, and our persona to those that are not so close.

Not long after I started working as a holistic therapist, someone came for treatments and a reading. By their vocation it could be natural to assume that they has a high spiritual EQ (remember assumptions make an ASS out of U&ME!). I sensed though that there seemed to be a dark energy (dis-ease) underneath this air of angelic perfection, she seemed so fearful. She was spiritually bypassing looking at her own toxicity and shadow, which over time she then projected onto me. Being somewhat aware of projection, transference and counter transference, I looked at my own energy and my own stuff, then had supervision on it. I didn't truly understand it and how I had been hooked in, for some years.

The true nature as you get to know the person will leak out. I often notice now if there are uncomfortable vibes underneath what someone is saying, it doesn't quite ring true; the use of a spiritual phrase which leaves me feeling uncomfortable, rather than blessed, or feeling sick or manipulated, or drained, because it doesn't seem real. It can be difficult to be honest and truthful with people when they are like that, because they have a strong defence against the truth.

This is where I came unstuck. She didn't want to hear what I thought I saw (fear) even though she had asked me. If this is the case, referral to someone else who is more trained to deal with this such as a psychotherapist or supervision can help, in order to identify our own blindspots too - and our shadow. Supervision is there to help support us as therapists, because it isn't very nice being dumped on at all!

This quote sums up spiritual bypassing *'If we put ice-cream on top of poop after a few spoonful's we taste the poop again. When we integrate negative traits into ourselves, we no longer need affirmations because we'll know that we're both worthless and worthy, ugly and beautiful, lazy and conscientious. When we believe we can only be one of the other, we continue our internal struggle to only be the right things.'* Debbie Ford.

## The persona

This is the part of us that is the ego, the false self, the mask that we put on the world, how we present ourselves in terms of what we believe others may find acceptable. It is the part of us that we have created in order to fit in. It is our less than authentic self, often where we are incongruent.

However, it can also serve a very important function, that it has helped us to survive. It is created in order that our needs in childhood, or adulthood, are met. When we are pleasing others, we are more likely to be fed, watered, clothed and have a roof over our head, etc. A part of us may have had to adapt in order to prevent or minimise abusive behaviour, so our persona or ego is our protector too and in that way has done a very good job.

At some point we may come to see that with compassion, the persona isn't always best equipped at dealing with certain situations, such as being a therapist. The breakdown of the persona leads us to realise that our perception wasn't 'real' and we begin to see aspects of ourselves in others that we may have judged.

There can be a sense of emptiness and life may not feel meaningful as this occurs. With that can come a sense of shame and guilt. As well as a sense of chaos, depression, confusion and even questioning of our beliefs and morals – all of which can be accepted and moved through when we practise self-compassion.

## Integrating the shadow

When we recognise the shadow within we gain strength and power from it, it no longer controls us, and we can respond to others with awareness, rather than overreacting. It is liberating to be able to say with complete acceptance and compassion for self, 'sometimes I can be jealous'. Admitting it and bypassing the ego can be the painful part initially as we allow ourselves to go into that darkness, but acceptance and compassion of why we are jealous or 'it just is as it is, we are human, we all have flaws and this is one such...' can allow us to let go. Understanding then helps us to process or 'digest it'. This gives us great strength!

Shadow work is fortifying, it helps us to own our flakiness! Very importantly, remember your humour, but also remember that there is never a truer word said in jest – this could be your shadow! But above all be kind and compassionate with that part.

## Do no harm

Whilst doing some counselling training, someone said to me 'you know you could dump your own issues on clients, because of your mental health problems?'. I understood projection, which is the process of 'dumping', and I explain more about it below. I'd had a lot of counselling and psychotherapy over the years and was aware that this was something I obviously wanted to avoid, with my premise of 'do no harm'. Upset, I spoke to my tutor about it, who asked, 'do they have experience in this area?' No, they didn't.

As I reflected on this, I remembered how I would rather see a therapist, who has been through and is actively working on overcoming their issues themselves. Direct experience can often open us up and every therapist has their issues. This, importantly, is why counsellors and psychologists have supervision, and also why I believe others therapists such as holistic therapists could benefit from it too. Whenever we are in a therapeutic relationship with another, a process occurs in that interaction and the key to a good session is keeping the client safe.

It is when we think that we are sorted and 'on it', that we have no issues, that we can make such judgements of another. We can then project our own stuff onto them. I had been aware of my own projections on others, but not so canny about people projections on me and this was a classic dump! Watch out for those moments of feeling superior or glib towards another, it can be a ripe time for us to be dumping our stuff on another - and also those moments where we may feel 'cut down to size', a gut drop or suddenly feeling tired or drained can be a sign that someone has dumped on us.

## Projection

Noticing when we or someone else is projecting can be a very freeing experience and a great facet of self-care. Understanding it helps us to protect ourselves better, so not to take on board another's negativity. Importantly, it can also help us to take responsibility for our own so that we don't dump it on another.

Have you ever felt dumped on? Maybe you felt cut down to size as I've mentioned, or confused and couldn't understand what the person was talking about when they accused you of something? This confusion can be an indicator that something is being dumped or projected onto us, we may feel squashed and it's usually because they are talking about their own issues and attributing them to us instead. It is like we are acting as a mirror for them, yet they aren't aware of their own reflection.

Much of the time we see or view the world through our own eyes as a result of our own experiences and beliefs, and we have tinted lenses through which we see the world. We may empathise and walk in someone's shoes but it's still our feet in their shoes. So put simply, whatever comes out of someone's mouth probably says more about themselves and their own experiences (and that includes what we say to others too). There are very few people who have such a high degree of self-awareness, that they are able to put themselves aside and see another in a truly pure light without the tinted lenses of their own experiences.

When I hear someone accuse, condemn or judge anyone, I now listen to exactly what they are saying and to what degree. I appreciate they are probably talking about an aspect of themselves that they aren't aware of. They may exclaim about another 'that person is so rude; when maybe they were being assertive or truthful. Yet they perhaps don't notice how rude they are themselves!

## Intuiting the shadow in another

Listen to the first thoughts that come into your mind before someone says something about themselves. I believe you can discern a book by it's cover. And that can guide us on how to interact with that person, which can be the ultimate form of self-care. When I was in psychiatric hospital in my early twenties, a patient walked past me in a corridor and my intuition screamed something offensive. Given that I don't usually have such strong negative thoughts about people (I saw the good, my shadow was rather repressed) I noticed this. Later, they sat nearby as we were waiting to see the psychiatrist. I asked a question and the reply indicated that this person was arrogant and pompous.

A few days later the patient came over to talk to me and was completely different. Their gain was my self-doubt. Immediately I dismissed the previous thought I'd had of them. I could see the person's energy then, though I didn't realise it was that at the time. A blackness seemed to surround them (this is the aura and energy if you are realising that you may have seen this too) Immediately, as they were now being nice, I thought that I was wrong. That was a huge stepping stone moment to look back on, in order to help me at a later date to know that I did have a good intuition. We can 'discern' a book by its cover. Pay attention to your intuition (see that section) as it can help you to notice the shadow of another.

But why have we attracted them into our lives? As I will explain in the next section, he was mirroring my own nature towards myself perfectly, but I didn't know that at the time. There is a saying that someone in a relationship may only treat you slightly better than you treat yourself. I realise now that given his nature, it reflected just how harsh I was on myself. I was in hospital having tried to kill myself, which is the harshest shadow possible. It wasn't until many years later that I could understand and begin to release my inner Sergeant Major from duty and cultivate a more kindly compassionate nature towards myself. When we begin to behave more kindly towards ourselves, and get more honest with ourselves, cultivating loving kindness, we are less likely to tolerate the cruelty of another. Natural boundaries form as we begin to see that this isn't acceptable.

## The mirror

Other people in our lives work like a mirror for us to see ourselves and we them, once we understand this concept. The mirror is where we can begin to see and own our own projections. What we see in another is likely in some way true of us too. However, we know that mirrors that we look at our physical reflection in can all be a bit different and can reflect back different things and distort others. On a psychological level, what we see in others can also be reflected slightly differently or distorted but the essence or overall being may be familiar in some way and once we understand it, recognisable for us.

So for instance if we say that someone is a psychopath, with the mirror technique it may not be a true reflection that we are a psychopath. However it could be saying something about us is similar, a bit distorted, but not literally. Pychopaths are known to lack empathy, and it might be that we lack empathy towards ourselves, we may treat ourselves very harshly. We may see a murderer and condemn them with venom, then when we look in the mirror realise that although we have never actually killed anyone, we do have a murderous desire to wring the ex's neck! Anywhere that there is judgement and lack of acceptance, our shadow may be lurking.

## Examples of our shadow exercises

Think of a famous person, real or fictitious who is a villain, write down some of their qualities.

Now ask yourself, what is that person mirroring back to you? 'Everything that irritates us about others can lead us to an understanding of ourselves,' said Jung. We like to demonise the villains, so we can dump our own stuff there, they make us feel better about ourselves, this is the joy of a baddy! So what happens if you empathise with the villains? This is NOT to condone their behaviour, but by seeing that a famous pop star is arrogant and irritates me, I was able to see that arrogant irritating part of myself, breath into it, accept it, I could then have compassion for that part of me that was trying to get it's needs met, and work to change or modify the behaviour if needs be. Then I can also be less judgemental of this famous person too.

When you last felt irritated, annoyed or experienced an emotional reaction to someone is it a reflection of anything you may have disowned within yourself?

If a part of you that you dislike rears its head, do you push it away or try to seal it off by saying that 'you weren't feeling yourself', or 'you were drunk', or 'you didn't mean that'. Maybe it is a part of you waiting to be owned - and it's ok (as long as we apologise for our misdemeanours!) Remember, we are human, none of us are perfect.

## Sitting in the dark

The beauty of the shadow work is that when we sit with our own shadow, we also become more accepting and less judgemental of other people's shadow and less drawn into the melodrama of experience. It becomes more a process whereby we become a 'silent witness' to what is unfolding or occurring. It is, as I have said, highly transformative but can be painful. Mindfulness techniques can help, as well as support from trained therapists. The process can be quite simple and there are a few approaches.

Using the mirror approach as I have mentioned, take the attribute and saying kindly and non-judgementally, 'I can be lazy', just noting and observing the feelings in our body, remembering that they will pass. Breath into them and reassure yourself that it is OK. Obsidian is a crystal which can be used for this work too. Either black or silver sheen (which connects to the soul too). This might help to focus our awareness of our darkness so that we can shine the light on it. As we sit with the feelings and emotions, owning who we are, just allowing the feelings to pass as they will (see the chapter on meditation). Remember that it's always darkest before the dawn, that these attributes have kept us safe and protected in some way and have served a purpose. Perhaps laziness was a protective measure against someone (another or yourself!) who wanted you to be on the go all the time. Indulging mindfully and with awareness in that feeling may be quite cathartic. You may notice a sense of relief and release as the energy fades and dissipates as it loses its control over you because you aren't judging it anymore, Often there is a feeling of being freer and more empowered in knowing who you truly are. Afterwards, do something nice for yourself - take especially kind self-care.

## The burdens that we carry

People who are over-giving tend to have a skewed sense responsibility. I believe that taking too much responsibility can literally pull energy from someone else, which we take on board energetically. Shoulder issues holistically may be related to 'the burdens that we carry'. If you have aches and pains in them you may notice that this is an area where you are affected. We don't always notice where things are playing out for us on a mental level if 'we just have to get on with it'. Our body then does literally carry the weight of the world on our shoulders.

For a while I'd been having a few minor issues with my shoulder so began working holistically in that area by having massage, osteopathy, and Reiki over the weeks to see what emerged for me mentally and emotionally. I started to realise at a deeper level and catch myself more when I would feel the sense of duty or guilt or responsibility to do something for another.

Unbeknownst to me in a friendship, because I wanted to help and support my friend, I started to wear myself out. Even knowing what I know about burnout, it slipped under the radar as often the learning curve highlights! Because I really enjoyed spending time with my friend and I was enjoying our friendship, I was over-doing things automatically. It had triggered my old stuff. She didn't ask me outright to do as much as I did do for her;  I wanted to. This can often be about our own unfulfilled needs, how we may sometimes do for another what we wished we'd had for ourselves. Have you ever wished that someone had been, or would be there for you?

When her needs increased for various reasons, I felt overwhelmed and went into shut down. I'd been experiencing a flare up of fibromyalgia, so my health had not been as good as it had been for a while and that had crept up on me. Very unusually for me, I'd started drinking more alcohol than I'd done previously; not much, but it was very unusual for me. I'd put it all down to a different stage of life, a life change, I was enjoying alcohol a bit now and relaxed and settled in my life.

As I contemplated my - and her - shutdown, it suddenly hit me, could you have a co-dependant friendships? I knew the answer, and googled it and I realised that this is what had happened. I realised I needed to take a step back, from that friendship and some others, to sort out what were my responsibilities in friendships.

## Projective identification

During some counselling training I sought to try to find more rational explanations for energetic transitions that seemed to be occurring 'psychically', between myself and others. On one occasion when I'd gone to take some water into the lounge, where my ex-partner was sat, I turned the stereo off. My ex asked me why I'd done that, I was busy cooking tea so had no idea why I would have done this, but they said they'd been just about to do that. On another occasion I noticed that I'd be in a good mood on waking but go downstairs and immediately feel irritated like I wanted to dig at my ex. I managed mostly to control it, and would verbalise anything that was appropriate, but came to realise over time and as events unfolded that it often seemed to be related to something that was going on for them.

I came across projective identification; the theory, suggested by psychologist Melanie Klein, that when someone is not 'owning' parts of themselves, because for instance they find that part intolerable, they can insert it into another. For example, the belief that 'I'm not a dispassionate person. I'm kind and caring' disowns the aspect of dispassion which can then be inserted into another person. It can sometimes be referred to as 'acting out', whereby the other person may find themselves acting out of character or in ways that isn't always usual for them, or at a level that seems out of proportion - an overreaction. So the person who doesn't want to own their own anger may find that they are attracting people towards them, who are angry and display that, until they see that they have unowned anger and stop attracting people into their lives like that.

Asking yourself if something is a pattern for you may highlight whether there is some shadow aspect at play that others are acting out around you. For instance, I kept attracting people into my life who were bullying in nature, because of my inner tyrant! By learning to sit with that, owning my inner bully to myself and others, understanding where it had come from and why and feeling remorse for having done that - but not beating myself up for it - helped. I then attempted to cultivate a more compassionate approach towards myself generally, which is still a work in progress.

I found it odd that I didn't miss my friend as I thought I would, my health started to improve again - and I didn't feel like I wanted a glass of wine as often. My friend struggled with alcohol. Without any blame on her part for my own behaviour, I wondered if I had absorbed part of this? I was mindful of whether I was blaming her, whether I was projecting my issues. We are complex beings and I believe that it is my responsibility alone to learn how to properly close the door to another. I realised that when we had been friends I had been thinking about her an awful lot, hoping she was doing ok and concerned for her. I'd left the door open to sponge stuff and take it on board. In not understanding where my responsibilities lay and maybe taking on some of her disowned responsibilities, I had tired myself out and also taken a part of her on. Are there any similar patterns in your own life?

I looked at other friendships and with those that were showing a similar pattern I stepped back to give myself some space and time to contemplate why I felt overly responsible. I went back to looking at shadow work. Sometimes we may benefit from taking certain issues to therapy and this I did by trying out my long desired process of Equine Facilitated Therapy.

If you've made it through this chapter, well done! I know I have found it particularly heavy going to write. That feeling is a good reason to practise Energy Hygiene, which helps us to shed heavy energy that comes up and out, as well as a healthy dose of self-compassion in the next chapter! Remember, once we emerge from the shadow we come out into the light; it's always darkest before the dawn and that through that process we can come up smelling of roses!

# Chapter Six

## Self-Compassion

### Compassionate self-treating

Compassion for ourselves is a more recently acknowledged and recognised aspect of self-care. Again, if we are speaking about the dynamic of over-giving, wounded healers and all the obstacles we encounter there, self-compassion could likely be a very large component part of our self-care for many of us. It has certainly been a large factor for me. Although I am not religious I enjoy aspects of various faiths and Lent is one such practise that makes me think. Several years ago I decided that I was going to give up being hard on myself. I am still joking that it is ongoing! And in seriousness it is. There are layers to being hard on ourselves. Our awareness hides in the darkest of places and pops out every now and then reminds us that the work is ongoing! Metta meditation is the practise of loving kindness meditation that focuses on love for self or another, for example breathing in kindness and breathing out anything that is unsettling us.

As I began to write this chapter, born of the question, 'How am I going to really deal with that deep doubt in myself, that is holding me back?' that emerged; it is interesting that on editing and working on the shadow section, it emerged again. It has been highlighted as the process of self-care for acceptance and a dose of compassion. This, as I've said elsewhere, is the key to a lot of my work and beliefs, we teach what we need to learn, that journey takes us to deeper understandings. Others who have written books are probably on some level talking to themselves too, as I speak more about in the section on symbolism.

So whilst humility and humbleness can be peaceful qualities, self-doubt can be damaging especially in the form of self-sabotage. Developing compassion for ourselves is different to pity, though that is still valid, a short spell of feeling sorry for ourselves can invite compassion in. Compassion directed inwards to self is a greater healer in helping to accept and allow what is happening, which can then naturally gravitate towards packing up the pity party and moving on to something constructive to work towards in our healing.

## Best-friend yourself

In any given situation, when you are struggling, what advice would you give to a good friend of yours? How kindly would you be? How compassionate would you be?

Compassion involves empathetic feelings towards ourselves but a component of that compassion may be the acknowledgement of our suffering. We can all too often dismiss ourselves, put ourselves aside and say 'get on with it, pull your socks up'. Would you say that to your best friend? Nowadays, I'd sack them if so! Self-talk such as 'I can see how sad and tragic that was for me' can allow us to feel the emotions, how deeply we have suffered, which can then allow it to dissipate and let go of it. As emotions emerge, we may shed tears and feel grief at our loss whether that be of a person, a pet, or of innocence, faith or trust, We nurture our own hearts when we best-friend ourselves. Like the shadow, we hold on to that which we cannot acknowledge. The only way out is through, otherwise it's still there lurking in the background until compassion shines its light.

## Compassionate self-talk

Instead of saying that we are stupid and berating ourselves with a horrible self-deprecating attitude and energy if we make if we make a mistake, we may instead say 'I didn't mean to do that, I'll have another go' or 'It's ok, I'm still learning'. If a friend turned round to you, like my colleague did years ago and said 'no, stupid!' what does that say about themselves as a person? They are projecting their own stupidity of attitude - as we are too when our self-talk is mean! Let's get wise with compassion. We really do owe it to ourselves, for that is how we come to value ourselves. Think about that. We really do owe it to ourselves, for that is how we come to value ourselves.

## Failing miserably or peacefully

With negative self-talk we may become miserable on top of what is already happening in our lives. I have an ongoing issue with sugar. Having given up smoking, lost a considerable amount of weight and endeavouring to keep it off, I find a mindful and intuitive approach to eating helpful. I still love sugar, I still love cake; it's also been a large part of my identity as most that know me know how I love afternoon tea! I coined the phrase 'sconisseur', such is my love of scones and my passion for rating how well they are made (in my opinion). However, I also know that my sugar consumption is above the recommended amount and it does have adverse affects that would benefit from some fine tuning.

Were I to give up sugar I am sure that my health would benefit, possibly not considerably, but enough to make a difference. However, on commencing this book I wasn't in the right place to do this. Instead of taking a stick beating approach as the food police would (and which has never been helpful for me), I adopt a compassionate, accepting approach whereby I trust that my soul will guide me to making that change at a time that is perfect for me. Until then it might be that it is teaching me something more that I may need to learn, for the growth of my soul. Sometimes despite the best of intentions we just cannot do what we know would be good for us.

I remember saying to my GP years ago, that I wanted to give up smoking. I was on the edge of another crisis and he said quite wisely, it's probably not the right time. Why set ourselves up for failure? Better to wait until the storm passes or other things in our lives change. Often what can happen is that when we give up one addictive behaviour but do not take care of the underlying issue, it just transfers to another addiction. We may be able to replace it with something more healthy, such as an exercise addiction, but what then happens when we can't exercise because we have an injury? The underlying issue still 'eats away at us'. If meditation in many of its various forms, or journeying, or journaling, etc., hasn't allowed the issue to emerge to be dealt with, having counselling or hypnotherapy or some other therapy should be considered.

## A compassionate approach to eating

As it came up to my 'deadline' for wanting to finish the first draft of this book, I mused upon why I hadn't had any recent cake inspiration of what to bake. Usually an idea comes into my head, but it wasn't happening. I had also got to the point where clothes were feeling tight. My compassionate approach to slimming then unfolded. There are moments where it seems that things fall into place and are so much easier to do. We do all 'know what we should be doing' most of the time on a gut level anyway!

A couple of people had mentioned calorie controlled diets and I'd enjoyed using an app to do that some years back. Having just also been doing the part of a nutrition course which focuses on our daily recommended intake, I decided to take the universal hints and focus in that way again for direct experience. I hadn't really intended to cut down on sugar, but it has happened quite naturally as I've tuned into food choices at each meal, mindfully asking my body what I need and want to eat. I don't feel like I have had to resist in a way that makes me feel deprived and if I really want something I have had it. I've cut down generally and a baked bramley apple and raisins replaces my slice of cake in the evening. It's not been difficult, I can feel my soul peacefully 'containing' and holding me in a space where right in the lead up to Christmas, I know if I want to I can have a mince pie but don't feel that I have to.

On a soul level I suspect that making these changes which have helped me on a physical level undoubtedly may also be helping me to be more fine tuned in reaching my self-care goal, to just finish the book. It is a compassionate approach to weight loss. Conversely, over the last month if I have had a few days where I have mindfully wanted to eat foods which will take me over the calorific intake recommended for weight loss, because I have been accepting of that is how it is for that day, I don't have that approach of 'I've fallen off the wagon, I may as well eat everything in sight now'. Instead, with mindful eating and compassion, I am able to stay in each moment and say 'it is as it is, each moment is a new one, I've had cheese scones for breakfast this morning, I will adjust through the day if my body is ok with that too and have a less calorific meal later on.' It's so much more of a peaceful approach than the stick beating one.

## Self-l

Loving ourselves is very difficult for most people, certainly initially on a SC journey. One of the original self-care tips years ago was the advice to stand in front of a mirror and tell yourself 'I love you'. The idea made me feel nauseous, such was my depth of self-hatred, which is sad and hence the absence of 'ove' in the section title! There was no way that I was going to do it. Brain washing myself wouldn't work because there was a core of darkness within me that really needed eking out and working on. Yes that darkness did need loving, but that way seemed ever so artificial. Like 'ice-cream on top of poop!' and the denial of the darkness, and a 'carpet sweeping' attitude had caused the issues in the first place!

Part of beginning to love and have compassion for ourselves, is to acknowledge and be OK with our differences and find another way if the one suggested doesn't suit. Adapting people's ideas can also work well. So attempting to learn to like myself was a start. I'd stare in the mirror and sometimes not even recognise myself. Because I'd not felt much compassion growing up, that was a difficult concept for me to mirror back to myself. I also figured that there were things about myself I wasn't keen on and part of that could be a nudge to make changes.

## 'Kindfulness'

Initial steps may be learning not to be so hard on ourselves, dampening down that harsh inner critic by beginning to treat ourselves more kindly, or with 'kindfulness', which was a phrase I heard not long back.

Catching ourselves saying 'you silly woman' when we've made a mistake could be the beginning of letting that go and thinking of other responses that are more kindly towards ourselves. Instead of saying 'you silly woman', we could instead acknowledge to ourself that we are trying our best (well done!). We all make mistakes and we can learn from them. What can I do differently next time? That really is a kind, compassionate approach, something that we would say to reassure our best friend. It can be the case that as adults we need to re-parent ourselves. If we have difficulty with this, we may want to take it to counselling.

## Compassion quietens the mind

As I've mentioned elsewhere, my difficulty with driving was due to anxiety that I felt. In essence I was quite a confident assertive driver, however, I would envisage the bonnet flying up on the bypass (if I could even get on there without someone else), 'breaking down' (I laughed at the irony of that symbolism, because I could do little to control my emotions, I was barely functioning). I had panic attacks where I would have to pull over into the lay-by, I'd be shaking and my comfort zone got smaller and smaller.

I tried and tried! I kept challenging myself and trying to find ways through it. I had done some counselling training with the awareness that it would be one step further in helping myself (and it was comforting that so many other members also had their own challenges of varying degrees). I remember doing solution focused therapy, which I realised was quite similar to manifesting or co-creating our own destiny. We were asked to visualise the issue that we had as resolved, rather than focusing on the issues that had brought me to that place. The idea was not to try to guess how I would get there (literally!) but just focus on doing what it was that we wanted to do. I saw myself driving confidently, I felt myself feeling free doing it. It was wonderful! There was an element of trust that the way to this place, achieving that goal, would naturally present itself.

What transpired was a moment as I was driving when the old familiar battle of anxiety was raging inside me, 'I'm going to crash… say the car breaks down… what happens if I burst out crying again and I can't stop… I hate driving, I wish I wasn't like this….' My counselling training and meditative practises brought forth the compassionate, higher wiser self which spoke inside of me which said 'but you are, you are anxious, it is as it is, no emotion lasts forever and it will pass', whilst also giving myself a big dollop of self-compassion and importantly too, acceptance and breathing into it.

I was driving and yes, I was anxious. But by fighting it, I was disallowing it and it was causing me more anxiety. By staying in the moment with it, breathing and allowing it, feeling it and staying compassionately present to the emotion, I was doing the exact opposite of what I had feared. Often with anxiety we are trying to push that anxiety away, because we are scared that by acknowledging it it will make it real and it will be worse. But by its nature, the 'trying' to push it away can make it worse, because we aren't accepting the reality that something is out of balance - and it isn't always the actual issue that triggers it. There can be underlying reasons. By just allowing and accepting it, within moments it passed, I calmed. My confidence in driving and in myself, then grew and grew because in my immediate locality I then rarely experienced the anxiety.

Bypasses and motorways were still challenging me, places I didn't know and when there was lots of traffic as my anxious mind couldn't process what I was doing… and with that came the next challenge to stay present, accept, allow and breathe through those moments. It has taken me years to regain my confidence of driving (it wasn't helped over the years by having unreliable cars either) and I have still not reached my driving goals yet, but I have so much more freedom again and gratitude for that. So great dollops of compassion for the anxiety is the hug that is needed to dissolve it in my book.

## The compassionate reflection

The following illustration is my experience and what follows may not be true for all, but something that I uncovered as I worked with self-compassion. For years I had experienced dysmorphic response when I looked in the mirror, such as 'urgh, how ugly or fat you are!' and it was pretty difficult to overcome. Sometimes sitting with the feeling beneath that reaction and breathing into it and allowing an emotion can help us to move through it, rather than trying to push it away or silence it with platitudes.

It was like the friend who tells me I looked great yet deep inside I had this awful feeling that no matter what she said, it wasn't going to change how I felt. I needed to do this myself, as you can if you notice similar. It may also be done with counselling or other therapies and identifying it is a good start, you can congratulate yourself on that. Also, how sad it is that we should object so strongly to ourselves, again sitting in compassion for ourselves and adopting an attitude of curiosity, asking ourselves what the feeling is behind that, breathing into it, may allow something to emerge.

I realised, with deep sadness and self-compassion as I did this, that I'd internalised the looks of sheer and utter disgust from a few significant people in my life who had looked at me with that way whilst growing up. To be an object of disgust is a tragic feeling of rejection, especially when we are a child we don't know how to challenge the reality that this is a person doing bad things to a 'good enough' person. Often this is 'normal' to us, we don't know any different on a surface level though deep inside may feel something is not quite right. To survive the situation and get through it, we may begin to believe it and take responsibility and begin to think that there is something wrong with us. If we can change something about ourselves then maybe life will get easier and we will feel better and be accepted.

Looking in the mirror at myself, was a reflection of and a trigger for those internalised parts. The shame and lack of acceptance for who I was had become imprinted in my psyche. If this happens frequently over time it can embed itself into our consciousness as if it is us. In contrast, when we see a look of love on someone's face repeatedly, we can surmise that we are a' good enough' person. It's tragic when we don't have that and not surprisingly can lead us to be someone who seeks and longs for approval from others but can barely look at themselves in the mirror because it carries that facial reflection of someone else's disapproval.

This illustration is a good case for energy hygiene and using some clearing methods, or shamanic work (extraction), to allow that internalised part to go, if the realisation of itself alone doesn't shift it as it sometimes can. We can ask that the energy be 'sent to recycling', wherever it needs to go from the highest good, maybe smudging ourselves (see Energy Hygiene section). Since then, my attitude to myself in the mirror has gradually changed to one of compassion and now, more-so, of acceptance and appreciation.

## Compassion time

Is there something that you are struggling with? If a response is pretty strong can you give 'it' or yourself time and sit quietly with it and breathe into it and allow it to be as it is without trying to change it? I stay with the feeling, that internal voice and accept and allow, all too quickly we push these things away and move on. However, if we focus on that feeling, a memory or an understanding may emerge which can help us to let go of whatever it is that is troubling us.

Having counselling, holistic therapies or psychotherapy may well help to develop a sense of compassion towards ourselves, particularly if we haven't been cherished as children. We all need to be embraced in that loving hold of accepting energy, it is a vital part of our composition. I firmly believe that a good therapist will mirror that compassion back to us which has a therapeutic effect over time which allows us to bloom.

## Forgive me

How can forgiveness be part of self-care? If we have unresolved issues with others that cause us to feel bitter, ruminating on it, angry and resentful it can deplete our energy. I remember my counselling tutor saying 'who are we to forgive?' and I think that perspective is worth bearing in mind. I perceived that to mean that sometimes forgiveness can come from quite an arrogant, superior place - that to me might be more about false forgiveness, when people seem to say too quickly and dismissively, 'oh, I've forgiven them'. It may come from our head or our ego rather than our heart. And it might be because it is too soon, or that on some level we've bypassed the pain and pushed it under the carpet.

Instead, forgiveness may come about via a process of understanding what has happened to us and letting that go in a natural process of dissipation. In that way forgiveness isn't even an issue. If we look at the wrong doings that have been perpetrated and how that felt to us and maybe even what that has taught us we may even feel a certain amount of gratitude for the experiences. I certainly wouldn't be doing what I am now if I hadn't have had the experiences I have.

Understanding why something occurred may help, as long as it doesn't re-traumatise. For example, behaviours can be passed down the family or ancestral line. If family members are raising their children, with wounds of their own that haven't been addressed (for whatever reason), the trauma can be passed from generation to generation. That can justify the behaviour, but it doesn't make it alright or excuse it. Forgiveness is not about making excuses. It doesn't mean to say that it is right, but a reason for why it occurred. We may forgive the person, and even understand why it has happened, whilst still not agreeing with or condoning the behaviour. I also think it is about being able to be present with the person as they are in the here and now, especially if their behaviour has changed.

My Nana died without me going to see her, in my early twenties. I'd put a boundary in place when I was eighteen, after a particularly distressing episode, and I didn't wish to spend time with her anymore. At the time I did question how would I feel if she died. My sense was that I would be OK. When I heard that she was dying I didn't want to go and see her, but also didn't want her to suffer. I phoned the hospital and asked the nurses to just pass on a message to say that her grand daughter Emma had called, it wasn't to send my love or anything like that but an acknowledgement, in a human compassionate way, that she may be suffering and I hoped that were not the case. I chose not to go to her funeral.

Some years later when I began psychic development, during meditation to connect with spirit she came to me. She was the first person to come to me, and the last person I would have wanted to see if I'd consciously have thought about this! However, it was a peaceful process, I got the strong sense that she was saying sorry and I was saying it was ok. There were reasons why she was the way that she was, it wasn't right but it was how it was and there was a reassuring sense of peace that flowed. And it also highlighted to me that I wasn't imagining it, because had I been I would have wanted someone else to come through!

Sometimes when people die, we may feel that things have been left unsaid. Having had this experience and being a strong 'knower' in spirit and the afterlife, I think more detail of the bigger picture is revealed when we can take a step back out of it. The things that have been unsaid in life can still be resolved in spirit. Sit quietly and just imagine that the person that is there in your minds eyes and say to them what you would have wanted to say to them in life. Notice how you feel as you do this, and what comes to mind.

## Forgiving ourselves

When a friend of mine became more and more ill, I felt concern for him. He found it very difficult to go out, he'd had a very tough life and was suffering poor health mentally and physically. His self-care was diabolical, he just couldn't seem to help himself. In my concern and exasperation (I was mindfully in rescue mode, and thinking I knew best to some degree) I tried to push the boundaries to encourage him to come out and come round to mine, thinking that this could make a difference to his life to get out of the house. He got defensive, said I didn't understand, I'd overstepped the mark (the road to hell is paved with good intentions!) and he put the phone down on me. He died not long after that and it was the last time we spoke.

He was a good guy. I know in my heart as soon as I heard that he'd died that it was the way that it was. I was sad that we'd argued but I knew that he wouldn't have wanted me to beat myself up for our argument. It was the way it was and I felt the warmth of his loving friendship from spirit, and whenever I hear the song Spirit of Radio playing, I think of him and smile!

If you don't feel able to or ready to forgive, it might be worth forgiving yourself for that. Forgiving ourselves is a great act of kindness to ourselves. Accepting that this is how it is right now and we are working on it. We are a work in progress!

The spiritual aspect of forgiveness may be to ask the powers that be, whatever your beliefs are, to help you. I went into a place of stick-beating unforgiveness for a mix up that had occurred at work. I was witnessing myself being hard on myself, I was trying to forgive myself but I just couldn't seem to and I just couldn't let it go - despite all the breathing and smudging and grounding! It suddenly occurred to me to ask God for forgiveness and I instantly felt calm. I was quite surprised and pleased. When it happened again I did the same, with the same result. So now, when I can't seem to forgive or have compassion for myself, I ask God to forgive me.

I believe that God is a pure energy, that is loving, non-judgemental (the jealous God is the human shadow), that gives us free-will to make our own decisions and learn through our experiences. I truly believe that this energy of God is within us all and within everything, so whatever we worship (even science! I believe God created and is the big bang and science?!) is OK and will lead us back to that energy if we follow the many paths up the same mountain. At the core of every religion or philosophy is love and if we can practise love and compassion for ourself and others, and have that as our focus and guide throughout life, I don't believe that we will go far wrong.

# Chapter Seven

## Zap the Attitude

### Channeling our negativity

I think that we all have layers of negative thoughts and challenges that we plod on with in life and this has been another hard chapter for me to write. I have recognised just how hard I can be on myself over the years and I think many of us are; see Internalised Bully further on. As I said, several years ago I decided to give up something different for Lent and chose to give up being hard on myself and I'm still working on it! So, I have had to give myself an extra push to writing it as a tendency to procrastinate and avoid it was kicking in. This is what I mean by direct revelation! Sometimes I like that I am still experiencing and struggling with issues myself, in that it helps me to empathise with clients. It is the beauty of this journey, that I receive timely reminders and experiences which teach me or remind me how hard it can sometimes be to battle some of the things that we do battle.

So how do we self-care ourselves, and challenge those negative thoughts that pop into our minds and either stop us from doing things that we want to do or compound our misery in life? Sessions with a counsellor or psychotherapist, hypnotherapist, or other may help to address deep rooted negativity and opening up to seek that help, then engaging in it can be therapeutic in itself. I often notice that people feel so much better just for booking an appointment for a treatment, because they are being proactive. I don't mind what that is about, whether its placebo or other; if we find something that works, great. But where do those negative thoughts come from, what's that about and what can we do about them as part of our self care commitment?

## The ego

Often we think of the ego in relation to someone who has a big ego. They come across as arrogant, pompous, full of themselves, big headed, power crazy, proud, self-important, and so on. Not many of us like to think of ourselves in this way, so those aspects of the ego may get shoved away in a box, into our shadow, as I've said. We may go to the other end of the 'egoic spectrum' where we are fearful, doubting, blaming, jealous, resentful, angry, desire separateness (feeling or wanting to be different) chaotic and so on.

The ego is our persona, as mentioned previously. It gives us our identity and a sense of self. It is the part of us that tries to keep us safe, protecting us or getting us through life. It is constructed in that way to serve a positive purpose for us. Judging our ego for doing the best that it can, in the circumstances that we have found ourselves in, can be counterproductive. Our ego has developed as a result of those circumstances.

Our behaviour develops in childhood as a result of the feedback or mirroring that we get from our family, our environment and society etc. As youngsters, we are dependent on others to get our needs met such as food, shelter, clothing and protection and our goal is to grow. To meet those innate needs we cleverly adapt to the circumstances that we are in. This is in response to what pleases or is acceptable to those who will meet our needs. In effect we are moulded by what others want. It might follow then that the ego, and someone who 'has a big ego' or is driven or motivated primarily by their ego (rather than their spirit or soul), whether that be that they are 'big headed', judgemental or fearful etc., has experienced a lack of protection and felt unsafe in some situation or other, whilst growing up. The ego, to protect the person, is a shield and will often over compensate to defend against the perceived threat.

## Over thinking

The ego is the part of us that is the over thinker, whereby we may live in our minds or our heads, rather than in our feeling bodies. To protect ourselves, we may have cut off our feelings. To have allowed ourselves to feel those feelings in that moment may have been too overwhelming, so it is a good defence mechanism. However, we may come to a place in our lives where our lack of feeling becomes a block and we feel stuck. We may realise that something is missing from our life, that by living in our heads, we are not a heart centred, loving, fully rounded feeling person. Having compassion and gratitude for that egoistic part of us that does rear it's head and tries to keep us safe in certain situations and acknowledging genuinely that it has done a good job of that, can help us to lessen it's role and responsibility so that we can expand and soften into our soul or spiritual self. There we find that we are connected to others and gain that sense of love and community, rather than the separateness that the ego creates out of fear.

The ego's modus operandi keeps us in our minds and is the part of us that creates that downward spiral of negative thinking. It projects thoughts, and 'what if?' worries into the future, tells stories and holds onto the past, whereas the spirit or our soul is fully 'present' in the here and now. For example, a noise in the house startles you and you begin to create scenarios where a burglar has got into the house and is about to stab you, then steal everything in the house, let the cats out and they will get lost and have no mum anymore because you will have died, etc.

Our mindful nature, or soul/higher self, would hear the noise, suggest breathing to calm self down, notice the feelings of fear but not attach to them or judge them (they are as they are). It may suggest to phone the police, or cautiously look for evidence of a break in (in which case we find the cat has knocked a vase over and is as startled as you!). It may prompt you to make the choice to sit and connect with that feeling, just letting it be as it is until it subsides (the concept of impermanence, no feeling lasts forever), and calmness is thus restored. As we move into our heart centre, we cultivate an attitude of kindfulness and compassion towards ourselves, rather than the berating, critical approach that the defensiveness of the ego creates.

## Heart or head?

A measure of self-care and client care that I was advised about years ago is to ask myself in relation to any client (and other situations I am in), 'am I responding from my heart or am I in my head?' To be in our heart feels soft, warm, loving and compassionate; we are open. If I am in my head, I am closed, guarded, mistrustful, suspicious, defensive and perhaps triggered in some way. That needs to be reflected on, which can be done by sitting quietly and meditating and contemplating the feelings that arise. If that doesn't promote a deeper understanding or a shift, it is time to take it to supervision and/or go for therapy. On some level, painful as it is, that person is probably teaching me something about myself which can ultimately be enlightening.

During some Reiki development work with an excellent teacher, certain behaviours made me feel uncomfortable. I later had an ominous dream involving my teacher. In a subsequent session, during the cleanse or a 'clearing', it emerged into my awareness via synchronicity as well, that this system of Reiki wasn't for me. The energy I enjoyed was great, however it didn't feel the right fit for my beliefs and values.

## Ego death

I realised that much of this was about facing my fears. I felt that I had to communicate that I wouldn't be continuing with her. I received some upsetting comments and 'love and light' disappeared from the few email exchanges thereafter. She also showed her true colours on a message forum that had been a great place for my development, with some fabulous people. She lied about her identity, then tripped herself up. All in all not a great example, even though she was a good teacher of Reiki, but also showed me what not to do as well. It took me a good while to understand her lesson to me. I was judging the judgemental, she was critical of her husband and I was judging her and dumping my unresolved stuff on her, as she reminded me of someone from my past.

I guess on a spiritual level it was also a clash of egos. I couldn't have handled it differently, I would handle it differently now in that I perhaps wouldn't get (so) involved in the first place. I received spiritual guidance through it all, but it still hurt and knocked me and my ego. This can be what I know as 'ego death'. It isn't a literal death, but a layer of the ego cracks open and breaks down, to let more light in. It is a very painful process! As mentioned elsewhere, it's the death rebirth cycle; an initiatory experience where we learn to let go.

## The internalised bully

If we have experienced someone who is critical and controlling, bullying and abusive in our lives, particularly as children, over time their words begin to sink into our psyche. In order to try to 'work it out', we may then either act out the bullying and bully others or turn it inwards onto ourselves, which becomes the internalised bully. The term we are our own worst enemy, is indicative of this. It also means that because we are continually weakening ourselves with harsh self-talk. We may have a pattern of attracting other people towards us who reflect those traits back to us. People subconsciously pick up on and are drawn to other people's weaknesses, as do animals. Think about the term 'hen pecked'. If there is a hen in the flock that is in some way weaker, the others gang up on it and pick at it, sometimes to death. People can be like that too.

Recognising if we have an internalised bully, which may be just answered by noting whether you can be hard on yourself (often a perfectionist too) and forming some self-care strategies to tackle that bully and lay it to rest, could lead to self-acceptance and a far more peaceful life. Also we may be less likely to attract people towards us who are hard on us too. If we attract bullies, it may well be that we are bullying ourselves. Remember compassion, would you talk to your best friend the way that you talk to yourself?

# The negative thought catalyst to self-sabotage

'I can't do this, it's probably going to be something no one wants to read, after all this work is it worth it, I've only just started why bother..' My stomach dropped, I felt scared, I sat and breathed into the feeling and allowed it without judgement. I realised that my goal wasn't really about other people reading, it was about completing it. Having had many books on the go that are unfinished (as yet!) my goal as a large aspect of my own self-care was to work on finishing a book that I'd started. My goal was to complete. Completing releases energy and healing. So in essence, whether or not anyone wants to read it is not the focus or the aim. I have had to go back to that several times during the writing of this to push myself through, because the negative self-talk decided to then up the anti and say that it was probably quite boring as well, or complex and too heavy in parts and... it goes on!

It's probably fair to say that we all have negative thoughts. Deciding if they have validity and whether we need to make changes can help us to chose whether to work with them or reject them as old programmes. Also noticing whether they are based in reality in the here and now? Getting Melfish and practising self-care is really learning how to deal with those negative thoughts that pop into our heads which can stop us from doing things. It may be a repeated process, the thought that people won't be interested in reading a book ('that I've written badly'), isn't a helpful part of me to listen and pay attention to with regards my goal of finishing the book. It may in the future be based in reality, but in the here and now is what I am concerned with, so I notice it and push that thought to the side knowing that in the past it was only trying to keep me safe but I'm a big girl now.

Deciding how best to SC ourselves during those times can be trial and error based upon knowing ourselves, if we are honest with ourselves. So writing this, this morning, I did feel low. My plan to complete chapter by chapter wasn't working, as my mind went off into unfolding tangents and various chapters emerged simultaneously. This is how I write, this is also how I tend to clean the house. Whilst I can trust now with the house that it does come together at the end, I still find it difficult with my writing given the amount of book ideas that I've had and started but not yet finished. The crux of it is, I will probably need to push through this to see what is on the other side.

## Battling the demons

When we are overcoming a challenge, the nature of growth can be that our boundaries may well be stretched outside of our comfort zone. As I work through driving challenges, driving on busier motorways for instance, I have felt very scared but it was an opportunity to also remind myself to stay present, just keep breathing and work through it as I gain more confidence. Sometimes we can find that our soul is taking the lead and guiding us through certain scenarios to help us grow.

There have been a couple of scenarios recently whereby I knew it was poignant to push through. The 'Hero's Journey' is where we go into battle with our inner demons. It's often said that 'courage isn't the absence of fear'. On the way to my first session of Equine Facilitated Therapy, I left with plenty of time spare so I wouldn't feel rushed. I came across a road block, the guy informed me that he didn't know the diversion route, the block had just gone up. My heart sank and panic rose. I used my local knowledge to the best of my ability and took a guess at the direction. The sat nav did pick that up, but repeatedly tried to send me back down the road where I kept meeting with other road blocks along it - with guys sat there in their road block vans not really being able to direct me! I found myself driving down narrow potholed country roads and coming across roadsigns back to where I'd come from which began to seem more appealing! 'Should I just give up and go home?' I asked myself. Time was really ticking and the sat nav said arrival would be late. I don't like being late. I noticed I was beginning to drive faster, battling with hopeless 'where am I?' panicky thoughts and feelings as well as a soothing 'just carry on, but slow down' thought. Something inside drove me and kept me going, kept me trying, a quiet determination.

Sure enough, eventually I rejoined the road past the last part that was blocked. I had remembered to breath deeply to activate my calmness and calmed myself as best I could, I figured that if I was late, I was late so what, I'd done my bit and left early, events were beyond my control. I got there a minute or two late. Self-care is about challenging those negative thoughts if they are our negativity, and not an intuitive feeling. I found out later that sadly someone had been killed in an accident on the road.

And as we are growing, we may be pushed a few times out of our comfort zone in short succession. A week or so later as I was leaving to travel to Aberystwyth to start writing this book, it was raining badly. I didn't think too much of it initially. However, as the journey progressed I began to notice a lot of flood water which was at times coming up to either side of the road. Rivers that I passed seemed very full and surface water on the road started to become more frequent. I felt a knot of fear that I kept breathing into and then came upon my first decision. A queue of traffic were waiting to take it in turns on each side of the road to go through flood water of some depth. Would my little car be ok? I waited and weighed it up, noticing other similar cars going through safely. It felt like there was a flow within me to breath and go. I did it, adrenaline pumped through, I shook on the other side and carried on breathing deeply to reset myself. Until the next one!

There were about three more, then I came to another big pool of water over the road, where I was the car in front, on my side of the road! I didn't know how deep the water was, (understandable cautious) negative thoughts crept in but I noted them and felt in for my intuition to guide me. There was absence of a warning gut feeling to back up so it felt OK to proceed. A 4x4 truck was trying to turn, I let him do that so he could go in front and I could see how deep the water was. I followed him gently though. It was very scary, I've not driven through water so deep. I drove through each one 'with God, with the Angels, with all the other powers that could be mustered in that moment!' but I felt exhilarated that I had faced those fears and that challenge.

That scenario was a reminder of how some have said that in those situations it's the devil or dark forces trying to put you off. That may well be, but I tend to take the view that it is my responsibility to challenge my own inner demons and those I can fight internally. I find that each time I do that, it is a facet of SC, because it builds confidence. I do think we need discernment, not to be foolhardy, to weigh up situations logically for evidence as well as intuitively and with gut feelings. Sometimes we might not be ready, or have the right tools to battle those demons. As it is often said, it is choosing the battles and that is about right timing.

## You and whose army?

Asking for 'human' help and support can be one way of working through an issue that challenges our SC. I sent a text to my partner, saying how I was feeling about the negative thoughts that I was having that morning about writing the book. I reiterated at the end that I'd realised my goal was to complete. He reassured me that everyone has doubts and sent another text following up about his faith in me that I'd do it. It reminded me in that sentence of how he has seen me face and overcome a number of goals and challenges since we've been together. I've grown and gained confidence as a result. So he was my army for today, I still sat there overwhelmed, and felt fragmented but decided I did really need to plough on and push through, even if what I was writing was coming out in tangents. And as I worked through the day, I churned out a lot. There are some ideas that may help others, but if it only helps me to complete my goal, my world will be a better place and in that I can radiate my own stardom within (which may spread out in a nice glow of self-confidence to reach others). Allowing ourselves to be supported and cared for by others can help us through.

## An attitude of gratitude

Cultivating the attitude of gratitude for the things that we have in our lives can be another great self-care tool. It can help to overcome depression and negative self-talk. I don't think that we should minimise circumstances in our lives by saying people have it far worse than me, full stop, because we are then not acknowledging our own suffering and noticing how we feel or paying attention to ourselves. It might even be the case that we are assuming that someone is suffering because we wouldn't like to live their life, yet they may cope with it fine, sometimes we just don't know! Twice in the last few days a different person has gone past in a wheelchair and two different observers have remarked to me, 'gosh aren't we lucky'. I contemplated why this had happened twice so close together, what was the message? It struck me. Are we assuming that those people are unhappy and suffering? We compare our awareness of what loss of walking and speech and so on would mean to us in our experience, but it might mean something entirely different to that person with the disability. Who are we to say or assume how another copes? They may well be very happy in themselves but again I can't assume.

However, what I also saw was that attitude of gratitude and what it meant to those people who were commenting and they were saying that they were feeling grateful for what they had. When we hear about the difficulties that other people experience, it can put things in to some perspective and enable us to think there by the grace of God go I! But is this true gratitude when we compare ourselves to another? I don't know. I muse that pure gratitude is perhaps when we appreciate within ourselves what we have now in the moment, perhaps compared to what we didn't have in the past. So I could say that today I am very grateful for the peace and quiet in my home where I am able to write and that space within myself to do so.

In a culture of more, more, more, sometimes we may have more than we are giving ourselves credit for or acknowledging. When I was really struggling to pay the bills due to ill health, I was able to see that at least I had a roof over my head and I was very grateful to my uncle for that. It didn't make it easier for me with regards paying the bills I still had to face and acknowledge that, but I could be grateful for what I did have. I also think that this is something that only we can decide for ourselves. To say to someone else 'be grateful for what you have' can show a lack of empathy and be counterproductive by minimising their experience.

When we have gratitude, we value what we have, we appreciate it and we connect better with the Universe, the powers that be as well as other people such as those strangers that talked to me out of the blue. Thinking about how our food has got to our plate, sending quiet thanks to the truck driver who has driven our groceries to the shop, the farmer or the labourers, the animals that have given us food, and the people who serve us in the shop and so on. When we really think about all the input into something that has come to us, such as a bag of lettuce, the refrigerators to keep it cold and the maintenance workers and manufacturers of those refrigerators etc., etc., the list goes on. It is quite amazing and a great demonstration of how interconnected we are. I like to think that because we are interconnected and that energy follows attention (i.e. energy flows to where we focus) that in some way my thanks will come to that person who has done their job and thereby helped me to do mine. Because fuelling myself with lettuce benefits me, which in turn benefits my clients! The energy cycle!

When we recognise what depletes our energy and what nourishes or tops up our energy levels, we can start to make more discerning choices. Try noting five things that deplete you such as doing the ironing or food shopping and ten things that nourish you, for example washing your hair or having tea with a friend. Focusing on the activities that nourish you daily can help to balance the depleting influences on your life and help top you up. It can also bring forth much gratitude for life.

## Gratefully living the dream

There may come a time when you realise that some of the things that you wanted in the past are now coming to fruition in some way. As I was coming back from having a break from writing and clearing my lungs with sea air, a sudden realisation dawned on me that I was living my dream. As I walked and the Air BnB where I am staying came into sight, I thought about how I had sat in the garden as a child of about eight or nine years old and wrote 'the dancing donkey' on my Palitoy typewriter. I'd always wanted to write. Since then, over the years when I'd been so ill but carried on writing all those bits of books, I'd harboured the idea that writers go away to a log cabin or a retreat to write. I thought about how amazing that would be to actually be in a position to do that, to have the courage to leave home and be well enough, but it seemed impossible and how would I ever be able to afford it? Yet here I was, right here, right now, doing just that! Living that dream. Gratitude swelled in my heart as I said thanks and let my self really feel that living dream.

## Non attachment to outcome

Only a year or so ago I had let go of the attachment to the idea that all the writing that I had done would come to something being published. If it did, so be it, but I wasn't holding onto hope anymore. I was quite contented with my life as it is and wasn't sure I wanted recognition, esteem, attention or extra work that I anticipated might come from published work. With letting go, I was also all too aware that this is about creating the void that appears when we pull back and genuinely let go. We stop trying so hard (which pushes it away). If the seed is to germinate it needs the dark to do so.

Non attachment to outcome has been another facet of self-care which sounds slightly contrary of making goals and such like, but as the above illustrates can help to overcome negativity and I chat more about it in the meditation section. Instead of staying focused on a point in the future, 'hoping' that something will happen, and getting disappointed when it doesn't and feeling a failure, etc., etc., we release or surrender the 'wish', goal or desire to the Powers that Be for the greater good. Trusting in the process of life, we stay in the present moment and get on with life. We trust that if it is meant to be part of our greater plan in life, then so be it and the Powers that Be will take care of the details, we just have to show up when instructed. It is a fine balance between giving up on our dreams, which can seem rather despondent but more-so it comes more from a place of acceptance that we aren't really running the show, but do have a part to play. If it's meant to happen, it'll happen.

## CBT

I'm not a huge fan of Cognitive Behaviour Therapy as there can be a danger of suppressing, rather than allowing, which leads it to be a temporary plaster over a wound that needs looking at more deeply. It is successful in the short-term, but people may find that because the deeper work hasn't been addressed, their issues just get transformed to other issues, so the phobia of spiders may go away but several months later a fear of lifts may begin. However, the process does help us to become more aware of our automatic negative thoughts, whereas previously we may have just felt depressed. I previously had CBT therapy which didn't help me, despite a good relationship with the therapist. However it did give me insight into my thoughts and the practise of challenging those thoughts I was then able to use at a later date, after I started meditating. This I believe is more akin to the practise nowadays where it can be combined with mindfulness based approaches called MBCT Mindfulness Based Cognitive Therapy.

The basic idea is that by keeping a record of automatic negative thoughts, when we experience what is troubling us, we gain enough awareness to begin to find alternative thoughts to challenge the negative ones. So as in the example previously, the dysmorphic part of me reared its head as I looked in the mirror. Negative self-talk kicked in about my appearance. I halted the flow of thoughts (STOP!) and instead managed to switch to a more compassionate attitude towards myself where I looked at myself literally in the mirror more kindly without the disapproval. Instead of letting those thoughts of 'you look ugly and stern today, your hair's a mess...' etc. I noted them, didn't attach to them, didn't judge them. I allowed myself to feel what was going on in the background and underneath and it then emerged who they had come from originally (that was now my internalised bully). I sent myself some loving kindly vibes and that I was OK in myself, especially with a more kindly attitude.

## Introjects

Another aspect of our negative self-talk can take the form of what are sometimes known as introjects. Introjects are like energy that we have taken on and into us. They are the 'should's', 'oughts' and 'musts' that someone may have told us or suggested that we do. For example 'I should go food shopping' on a Friday night. When you find yourself doing this, ask yourself 'who says or said that I should go food shopping on a Friday night?' Is it something that as a family your mum always did, so you think you 'should' too and feel guilty if you don't?

Reevaluate whether you want to continue to do so or not. A common one is 'you must be quiet when you are in the library'. Many of us find ourselves whispering, but in our local library, the librarians will talk at a low, normal level. So things can change and our thoughts and thought forms may need updating too. On a more challenging level are the introjects that may have come from others, that have seemingly programmed us. If we have been repeatedly told that we are 'stupid', or some others negative comment, we may replay this in our mind too, taking it on as our thought without questioning it until it causes so much destruction or upset that we think to challenge it.

## Realistic thinking

Asking ourselves who may have called us 'thick', if there is any evidence for that and can we reframe it to something else can help us to move forward and let some of the past go. For instance, if we have never been good at maths and someone said we were thick, we may have carried that with us all our lives and even say to others 'I can't do maths, I'm too thick'.

Each of us have skills and talents, and weaknesses too. Reframing our inability to be good at maths, by just accepting that it is so and not a reason to judge ourselves harshly or unkindly, can be quite liberating. I realised that I would never be good at maths, I've never been told I was thick, but I was told that I wasn't good at it (I wasn't) and I had a tutor for years. No matter how hard I try to focus and concentrate, I accept that I won't ever be good at it and I will make mistakes. My skill is more with writing and therapies. So I let an accountant do my maths, accepting that it's OK. I'm not thick or stupid because I am not talented in that area. That act of self- acceptance helped me move forward in leaps and bounds with being self-employed, because when I first started out I was almost too scared to earn because it would create book work! I had to call on others to help me to assist me to move forward with that. So self-care can be getting yourself an accountant or asking someone else to do something that you can acknowledge realistically that you will never be good at. That isn't a negative thought, that is a realistic one.

## Self-care blockers

We may have to undo years of work where we have taken on board the things that have been 'introjected' or 'inserted' into us over the years, by family, teachers, society and also ourselves via our thoughts and beliefs, etc. Classic self-care blockers can be ideas such as the family values 'it is selfish to say no' or 'if someone does something for you, you owe them one'. We may then want to question those internal 'programmes' and see whether they need updating and reinstalling.

'I should be kind to others', 'Saying no to others is mean' and so forth can create internal conflict. These two sayings are very common blockers to our self-care! We can't bare to say no because we may feel that it hurts us too as we've failed (our parents or whoever told us this is the case). These beliefs sit within us creating a self-imposed prison, they keep us trapped.

Look at your own 'should's', 'oughts' and 'musts'. 'I must be a good girl because people will dislike me'. They are often generalisations. Some people will, some people won't and we can't control another's perception of us. 'Those that matter don't mind and those that mind don't matter' is a great way to counteract this idea. If for instance we perceive saying no is bad, then we doom ourselves, before we even get to the part where, 'some people might not mind and think it is OK that you said no. That person might need to learn to do it for themselves. They may be much happier in the long term if they could.'

As times change, so too can our concepts of what is acceptable or not. It is fortunately becoming more acceptable that it is counterproductive to give our all and many people are beginning to see that self-care is a wise way to go, rather than the old concept of running ourselves into the ground. The martyr is swift becoming history, and we are waking up to the understanding that had she been more aware she would have taken responsibility for herself at an earlier point!

# Chapter Eight

## Toxic Guilt & Over-giving

### Appropriate guilt

Appropriate guilt is where we mistakenly stand on someone's toe, we feel a sense of responsibility and upset at what we have done when we see the pain on their face. Immediately we apologise and seek to rectify our wrongs. It is justified that we feel we have done something wrong and the guilt diminishes when all becomes well again. With toxic guilt operating in the background of our consciousness as well, it is likely that we will overly fuss them and worry that we have really injured them, etc., etc.... and the etc's go on! Healthy guilt means that we apologise and move on. Toxic guilt may cause us to ruminate and hold on to what we have done, berating ourselves and being overly harsh towards ourselves. Healthy guilt helps us to be honest and truthful with others, we don't like to tell lies and feel guilty if we do. Toxic guilt may rear its head if we need to tell a white lie! (and question whether white lies are ethical anyway, that's another debate!)

### Nothing is ever good enough

As children, we may naively think that our parents or teachers intentions, because they are the adult and they know more, are 'right' and we can swallow their philosophies whole. Telling us that we are selfish or lazy if we don't give 110% sets us up for a lifetime of over-giving and guilt when we don't attain that 110%. We may have been compared to another person, a sibling, or someone else which highlights how our performance 'should be'. We start to think things like 'I should give 100% even if I'm worn out and ill, because otherwise they will be upset with me'. It can leave us with a sense of being very deeply flawed where nothing that we do is good enough and we can never be enough for anyone. We maybe caught up in a perpetual cycle of trying and people pleasing and may even be repeating the same mistake with others.

People who are so critical will never be satisfied unless they gain awareness and look to their own SC to rectify their own dissatisfaction in life, by learning to take responsibility and meet their own needs. Obviously it goes without saying that we are responsible for meeting children's needs. But in other dysfunctional scenarios, until then toxic guilt trippers will keep expecting others to make them happy and blaming them when they don't. Hence toxic guilt is born, that sense of being overly responsible for others wellbeing and welfare and never being able to be or do enough.

## Emotional blackmail

Educating ourselves on how others can be emotionally manipulative is a definite facet of self-care. 'If you loved me you'd do it', 'oh you never come to visit me', 'I'm so lonely I can't do anything'. The idea is that the person gets to avoid taking responsibility for themselves and feeds off others. By 'winning' they are then rewarded by getting them to do their bidding.

Guarding against emotional blackmail is a SC strategy and standing our ground firmly in doing so. Those who are 'needy' or 'manipulative', sometimes know as 'drainer's or 'energy vampires', will employ a variety of tactics to get their needs met. These can include pouting and pulling a sad face (sometimes done jokily when testing the boundaries), playing the 'poor me' victim, telling you that no one else can help, saying that you are the only one they can count on, that no one else understands them. They may try to make you feel special and idolise you, crying, ramping up the drama and exaggerating. Remember NO is a complete sentence. You do not need to justify. It's likely that this person has and will take and take and take without truly valuing you. The difficulty is emotional blackmail is hard to overcome and stand up against until you begin to value yourself and recognise your own self-worth.

## The birth of over-responsibility

During therapy, I realised that due to the circumstances in childhood, the only thing that I could control was my feeling of taking responsibility for the actions of others. By trying to work on myself to change, may also change what was happening around me. It is a coping mechanism and one in which I think many of us drawn to doing therapy work for others may have developed. Sometimes it is also called the identified patient in a family as well, where one person in the family takes on the responsibility for the issues of the whole family. Commonly also known as the black sheep! Many therapists are black baas.

Over responsibility goes back to the Caterpillar and the Butterfly story as we saw in the chapter Healer Heal Thyself. it may also come into play if we have experienced toxic guilt, emotional blackmail and have been manipulated by others. It can be a reason why we end up offering to do too much for others and draining ourselves. From my point of view there can also be a mild arrogance and superior part of me that might assume I could either do better, or they can't cope. Being

OK with accepting that is part of myself, is part of shadow work and that is an ongoing process of awareness, that I can be a bit of an interfering busy body too - read on.

# Over-giving

Over-giving is a depletion of energy. By it's very name it implies a self-draining mechanism in many ways but there can still be a payoff for us in some other way. Generosity is a beautiful quality, when there is no outcome attached to it, 'ooh they'd give their last penny away' is seen to be a good thing and something that some may aspire to when they take a vow of poverty, for example. To not be so attached to our worldly goods, possessions or time can be the sign of a generous hearted person. Who wouldn't want to be like that? How many of us would like to be perceived as the opposite, mean and stingy; a scrooge?

There maybe a secret need or a payoff for the giving though. Giving too much maybe an automatic reaction born out of feeling that we are not good enough, or sufficient as we are. We may not feel entirely worthy as a person, hence we give more to overcompensate for our perceived lack. It maybe characterised by giving too many gifts to others, people pleasing, being excessive, maybe manipulative, or feeling overly guilty in nature. It may come from having been overly criticised in which we attempt to please another by soothing or calming them in some way. It may be that we are over conscious of what another's need are, rather than paying attention to our own needs. Sometimes we may feel that it is expected of us, or it has just become our norm and an automaton.

I realised that I was not giving from a place of pure giving when I noticed that I felt like I needed to buy a relative a bar of her favourite fruit and nut chocolate. When I did that she was pleased and wouldn't criticise me as much, at least for a bit. I came to realise that this softened her. It was effectively 'buttering her up' and came out of survival mode, to make my life easier. As I realised this though, I felt that this wasn't really quite right, I shouldn't have to do that to be accepted or respected by her or others. My people pleasing behaviour was programmed in by then and I didn't fully understand the implications of it.

We can be over-giving in many ways, not just material items or gifts. When I wasn't working I often felt guilty about not being able to contribute financially to certain things, birthdays etc., but I felt that although I couldn't give materially I could give of my time. That came naturally to me. I would happily sit and listen to friends talking about their problems for hours.

## Over-giving time

When I first started working as a holistic therapist, I'd completed quite a few hours of counselling training. I could understand from that perspective the counselling hour and keeping to that time boundary, it seemed quite clear cut and straight forward. However, as an over-giver I got it in to my head that a holistic treatment, say reflexology, which was 50 mins and then the consultation was 10-15 mins and then time for them to come round afterwards and reappoint, etc., took another 10-15 mins. So, often, for an hour treatment, I'd be allowing and doing ninety minutes.

I started feeling overly tired again and knew something was amiss but initially wasn't sure what. I found myself a supervisor and my consciousness flagged up, with guilt, my over-giving of treatments. I calculated that by going over by 30 minutes, if I had 5 clients a day, 5 days a week, that was 2.5 hours a day I was giving away and 12.5 hours a week! I was giving over a day's work away for free every week.

It needed to change, but this of course brought up the concerns that if I withdrew my time and kept to the boundaries of 60 minutes including consultation, etc., clients might not like it and go elsewhere. I reasoned that possibly if I wasn't tired I would be giving a more focused, quality not quantity treatment and I just had to trust! It was quite scary and felt like I was taking a risk, but my intuition told me this was right to do. And so it was. To my knowledge, no one complained. My regulars carried on coming and didn't even really seem to notice! It also put the onus on the clients who may be chatty during the consultation, that over time they came to realise that their treatment would be shorter if they did that - which some of them don't mind anyway, if they like a chat.

## Stealing time

Many of us may also have been on the other side. Being a recipient of someone who is over-giving can sometimes feel like we are being bombarded with gifts or with overwhelming energy. It can sometimes feel like it's a bit 'too much'. A teacher that I had was an excellent teacher but continually ran late, often by about half an hour. She aptly commented one night that she was 'stealing time', a phrase I'd never heard before but reasoned was really quite true and even though I enjoyed the classes, it did feel like my time was being taken on a dark winter evening when I just wanted to get home. For others, that would, of course, be seen as a plus and desirable to be given that extra time, so it can work both ways!

What leads us to over-give in that situation? We may be under an illusion and like to think that we are giving freely and unconditionally of our time, that it is nice to give something extra. It may however be conditional, if we look at ourselves honestly and realise that we are gaining something from it, whether that be pleasure or even power from it for ourselves. We are being paid in kind, with attention or gratitude, but what happens when we don't get that or 'people aren't grateful' or don't go away and tell all their friends how wonderful we are? We are human after all and all have wants and needs which work themselves out in various ways. Do you enjoy what you do and that is your reward? It is hard to be self-less and very few of us may manage this. If we do, it might be that we do not rely on this for a living. It does become a different kettle of fish when that is so. If we are truly giving unconditionally, people can be ungrateful, not say thanks and it will not make any difference to us because there is no attachment to the outcome. We aren't looking for acknowledgement or thanks. I think truly unconditional giving are the things that we do for another without them or anyone else knowing about, such as leaving a present on the doorstep for someone and telling no one else. A need to share the good things that we have done, can mean a payoff for us with attention or flattery that we 'are good' people. Do the good deed and say nothing. Because few of us are at a level whereby we can give unconditionally of ourselves without draining, depleting or burn out, this is why we charge for our work.

If we don't get attention, thanks or gratitude, if we aren't learning anything for ourselves and we start to feel drained, it indicates that we could be over-giving and looking for a payoff. It may help us to look at our boundaries and the sense of value that we have for ourselves and our attitudes there which is covered in those chapters.

## Volunteering or charging for our services

Many people may start off in an area of work by volunteering their time. I found that by doing voluntary work for the cat rescue and by giving treatments freely through voluntary work, I gained valuable experience and in that I benefited, it was my payoff. However, we may find that we come to a place where we feel sufficiently experienced in whatever it is that we do and start to consider charging for our time, especially if we get busier and find that we have less time so notice we are depleting. Whenever I need to put my prices up, my energy levels start to flag. I don't like doing it, I am committed to try to provide a reasonably priced service in my job that benefits all, but I also don't want to struggle. Charging the right price is self-care!

Nowadays as I have more experience and more clients, I also have to be mindful of my energy reserves. I check in with myself to see whether I have 'spare' energy to do special offers, give away gift vouchers or time for charities and raffles and sometimes I have to say no, because maybe I need that time to give to myself.

## Perfectionism

This can be a major cause of over-giving as well as creating a deficit of or a barrier to self-care. Perfectionism is wanting something to reach an ideal or to go above and beyond that. We may have high unrealistic expectations of ourselves, which can be hard to maintain over time. A perfectionistic attitude can keep us stuck, rather than moving forward in life.

## 8. Toxic Guilt & Over-Giving

I had a client come to see me who was a self-confessed perfectionist. She'd bought some card making materials, but was scared to use them because she'd spoil them. I suggested that she take the first card out and purposefully make the worse job she could of it, mindfully make all the mistakes that she feared making, in order to let go. She came back to see me having really enjoyed herself and she presented the worst card ever, with glee, to her husband! Much to his chagrin I think! It allowed her to let go, and she was able to benefit from her hobby at last.

We can have rigid expectations of ourselves, such as 'a job isn't worth doing if you can't do it well'. It is a black and white perspective that is overly harsh and critical. It stopped me from moving forward for some years, believing that I had to give 110%, until I experimented with giving and doing a little less, I drew the reins in, stretched myself less and dropped down a notch and began to get things done. I still can resort to it, I have had to keep reminding myself whilst writing this, when I fall into default 'must include everything I know' mode that my goal is to finish this. My achievement will be in completing this, as part of my own self-care development. Anything else will be a plus and a bonus.

Staying in the moment rather than projecting into the future with worries may help us to let go a little. Thoughts were flashing through my mind as I wrote this of how, when I've done the rough draft, I will have to go back to it again. If someone else edits it and gives me other advice will I have the oomph to keep going back to it? Putting those thoughts aside, because they are depleting and won't help me get the book finished in the present helps. I will cross that bridge when I come to it, but for now here I am right now in the present typing away!

Perfectionism may stop us from engaging, and participating. It may make us feel rigid and inflexible, hemmed in and stuck. It may be that we fear others' opinions of us and overly focus on our shortcomings rather than the positives that we have achieved. A psychologist once said to me, 'what have we ever learnt by succeeding first time?' The fear of failure maybe so great. Cultivating some compassion for ourselves and learning not to judge ourselves so harshly can be a real relaxer of the perfectionistic attitude.

## Intoxicating guilt

Driving along in the car, at 30mph in a 30 zone when a police car comes up behind you, how do you feel? I used to feel a huge wave of guilt, yet I had done nothing wrong! It stumped me for years why my conscience seemed to be playing up this way and I put it mainly down to my anxiety. I'd wondered if it was linked with a fear of authority. It can often be linked with authoritarian parenting too. I came to realise over the years, that it is an excessive form of guilt, or toxic guilt, brought on by negative conditioning and then perpetuated as an adult by a harsh inner critic which continued to allow others to dump on me. The only thing that I was guilty of when the police car saw me was being under the influence of intoxicating guilt - it really does skew our perception!

Toxic guilt can cause us to be vulnerable to the wants and needs of everyone else but ourselves. It is centred in the solar plexus, alongside its companion shame. Like an ulcer, or a black hole, it can literally eat away at us until we silence it and close that gap, with firm boundaries and a stern 'no more'! Toxic guilt isn't a healthy way of relating to others and can feel like a sense of duty in overdrive. Alongside it, are the other faithful companions resentment and discontent.

When I think about toxic guilt, I get the visual image of inner blackness, like a dark energy, placed there by the needs of another who is manipulative. This can happen during childhood or as an adult, when we are excessively put upon, often by another who is not prepared to take responsibility for themselves. It is what I call 'dumped' energy - sometimes known as 'Wetiko' - as I mention in the shadow and energy hygiene. It is energy that isn't inherently ours. A therapy session with someone who works with energy may help to begin to clear some of this, as essentially it might be that we have become a toxic dumping ground for other people's stuff. And not only that, but repeatedly seem to call it in and attract people to us who will play on that.

So how does it happen? When we are repeatedly around people who criticise us, it literally picks holes in us energetically. We can absorb and take on those 'voices', into our own psyche so they almost become a part of us. It is like an energetic possession, until we come to realise that it isn't true and rid ourselves of those 'introjects' - see the section on Zap the Attitude for more of this.

## Over-takers

Sadly, I started to notice that I felt drained by a friend. I frequently felt guilty around her for not going to see her enough; she would make passive aggressive remarks such as 'it would be lovely to see you more often', and that statement in itself sounds almost like a compliment, however there was this tug underneath where I felt 'not good enough'. Fortunately others on this occasion did notice this too (we can sometimes doubt our own experiences as we are learning) . For anyone who has been on the receiving end of that tug, it is usually barely imperceptible to anyone other than who it is directed at unless they are aware of this process, because it is only directed at the person that they are attaching to as they take energy. More often than not this completely unconscious. It is about getting needs met and we all have needs. It was hard because she was elderly, and I had a genuine love for her, but it was draining our friendship. Her family didn't come to see her often and I wondered why that might be, if that was telling on some level. I often felt overly responsible; it can be such an automatic reaction for many of us.

Her demands of me felt too much with my own ill health and capabilities. It was a difficult pattern to break and to take a step back. I didn't know how else to break it but by seeing less of her, as with a recent friendship. We may sometimes have to repeat our mistakes a few times to understand the intricacies of where we are going wrong! Now I understand that I have had a habit of forming codependent friendships, I recognise at a deeper level that need for boundaries and strengthening those. Good fences make good neighbours. By understanding what is and what isn't our responsibility can help us in the process of releasing a predisposition (or a programmed one) to toxic guilt.

Those of us who are caring find this a very difficult concept to act on. It seems cruel and very very difficult to be withholding. However, sometimes that can create the space (the universe not liking a void!) and let someone move on to a better place. This was literally true of my friend as it transpired that she went into a nursing home and had the time of her life and lots of attention!

## Give the guilt trippers another map!

Toxic guilt can lead us to say yes to every request that is made of us, sometimes without even thinking whether we can or if it's convenient. It is tied up with a sense of being overly (and irrationally!) responsible, as well as shame for not being enough. Learning to say no or taking a step back is a challenge, and it does involve us sitting with some uncomfortable feelings initially, but can be done! The beauty of it is allowing time to pass and seeing that things tend to come right anyway with or without us. We may come to realise, ironically, that we really aren't the be all and end all, we don't have to save the world as well as all the guilt trippers as they may quite easily and very quickly sort themselves out anyway, They seem to have a habit of landing easily on their feet, or find somewhere else that they can get their needs met and we realise that we really weren't all that in the first place! This can be a real relief, as well as energy conservation. That's one app that has been running in the background that we can stop so that our battery doesn't drain as quickly. Give the guilt trippers another map so that they can go holiday somewhere else that isn't at your expense.

Are you an interfering, fussy, know-it-all, busybody? Yep, me too sometimes! Been there done that, still sometimes find I've got that t-shirt on! This idea of how we should help others when we see a minor struggle instead of letting the person do it themselves and without them even asking for help, can be invasive and even detrimental for many people, if it creates a dependency, rather than being helpful.

Because of my reactions to my programming, I had always assumed that everyone needed or wanted help. As my own independence has grown, I know that I can feel a bit smothered when people rush in to do something for me that I would rather do myself. I feel my energy can drop and this can indicate that the other person is gaining energy from me, and it might be that they (myself included) are doing something for another to make ourselves feel better on some level. A need to be needed is common.

This need can also come across as a bit of a put-down, even if not intended. For example, someone assumes that the person can't do it themselves, with a thinly veiled, 'I am better at this than you are'. This can sometimes be noticed when people tell you how to do your job! We may then characterise the person as ungrateful, if they don't show their appreciation for something that they didn't even want in the first place! We may wonder why we are tired and burnout, having given all our own energy away helping others, who didn't actually need it anyway. What a waste! It's like having the central heating on, leaving the windows open and wondering why our heating bills are so expensive - what we can aim for is energy conservation. I like the angel's approach which says that they can only help us if we ask - unless it's life threatening. So with my busy body helping ways, I try to remember this too and hold back.

Giving unsolicited advice can give people a sense of power - because they are often sourcing it from us! Have you ever felt that slighted feeling when someone starts to hand out advice that you actually didn't want? The difficulty with over responsibility can be when someone is throwing us hooks and we are there with bated breath - what a great recipe for depletion!

# Hooked in

This can happen when someone is a perpetually complaining about their lot, that they have a lot of drama going on in their lives and through those complaints are inferring that they want or need help with something, instead of directly asking. Almost knowing that principle that the universe hates a void, if they complain about that deficit, maybe someone who is a classic over-giver and just waiting to jump into that void will fill it!

If we are good fisher people we may pick up on those hooks and find ourselves getting reeled in to a never ending depletion of energy! Thinking that we are helping we may offer suggestions. To give a good example, the common cold is a favourite one, someone has a moan about it - saying they feel awful, seemingly sounding like they would prefer to feel better and everyone replies with their favourite remedies that help them and suggest they try this or that. It may seem like unsolicited advice as they may not be directly asking for help, but there is that gap or inference there that draws us in.

Every suggestion that is made to the person, is returned with a reason why they can't do it. Instead of being honest or able to say, as some now will - 'I just need a moan, I don't need help or advice I want a pity party, please send me a hug or some energy thanks, then I will pack up and move on with it!', it feels like we are being played as we search ever deeper into our treasure chest of home remedies for colds. They have us hook, line and now also with a stinker cold as we are worn out too! The continual repeated negativity, if this is a pattern for the person, can deplete us too. They can wear us out, IF we allow it! It's the 'energy vampire' scenario and you will very rarely hear of them finding solutions that have empowered them or taking responsibility for themselves, 'I feel rubbish so I am just going to try some eucalyptus oil, has anyone else got any good suggestions?' Give them an inch and they take a mile.

Take a step back, walk away, remember the angels. Remember energy conservation. Remember you matter too, value yourself and your energy, you need it. Toxic guilt and over-giving has no place in replenishing your batteries, however letting them learn to do for themselves can ultimately be the best thing that they have ever done for themselves. Like the butterfly they may literally fly.

# Chapter Nine

## Boundaries

*"At 70 years old if I could give my younger self one piece of advice, it would be to use the words, 'f$@k off' much more frequently."*
*- Helen Mirren*

## What are boundaries?

Boundaries are the invisible line that we draw around ourselves, consciously or unconsciously. This communicates to the other person where they end and you begin. It is the space that we have around us, on a mental, emotional, physical and spiritual level. If our boundaries are invaded we can feel exhausted, violated, injured, scared, overwhelmed, irritated, angry and frustrated. When others take continually from us, it can be draining. Communicating our boundaries is our responsibility to ourselves, however identifying when our boundaries have been overstepped can sometimes be difficult to spot, as it maybe very subtle or normal for us to be trampled on.

Tuning in to our own feelings and emotions when we are around someone may be an indicator, if we are in tune with our feelings. We may notice feelings of frustration, resentment, irritation and tiredness. We may just not want to be around that person but we might not really understand why if we don't understand the concept of boundaries. If we have been raised with poor boundaries, we may have to relearn about identifying our space, what is me and what is you, what we are responsible for and what we are not responsible for.

Boundaries can be too close or too distant, they can be rigid or too flexible. A healthy boundary is somewhere in the middle of those factors and will vary according to who we are with. For example, those that we trust we open our boundaries up to, dysfunctional others we may keep more of a distance from Like the castle walls, boundaries are there to keep us safe and protect us. There is a saying, good fences make good neighbours.

## A safe container

Boundaries can be a safe container; therapeutically, a means of holding ourselves - or others - whilst we heal. Within those boundaries we give ourselves space to process, time-out, a rest, a re-charge so that we can come back to what is us and find ourselves or re-align ourselves. Many people find that as part of their personal development journey they may need to make more space or distance themselves from people who either lack self-awareness or are toxic. This can be a very difficult decision to make, but can sometimes come down to a black and white choice, 'it's me or them', if our health on some level is suffering too. Having that 'space to breathe' can reorientate us, come back to ourselves and reset us.

## Boundary lessons from starlings

Taking a break from writing, I went for a walk to watch the starlings murmurate. As I walked, the subject of boundaries came into my mind and thoughts flowed. If you have ever watched the starlings murmurate, as they flock together in a huge swarm they seem to pulse, they twist and turn in unison, seemingly connected. The idea behind them doing this is theorised to protect or distract predators, it may well be part of it, but I like to think there's something more. As I watched them this evening they spoke to me of community. A flock of them pulsed together, then as a smaller flock came to join them, they moved to them to gather them in. They did this repeatedly, and I wondered about the social aspect, just as there seems to be when the red kites gather at a feeding station.

When I've watched them before it has looked like a pulsing beat of togetherness and as a lady also watching them said: 'the one mind'; they do move as one. Apparently they watch the closest seven around them. I realised as I watched them that they need to manage that space, that boundary around them, otherwise they would crash. Too near they would collide, too far the system shatters and separates, as it did at one point. They broke into two distinct separations as if a shock wave had gone through them (there was some sort of noise) and one of those separations also separated (a bit like the fragmented self!) This is very true of boundaries, too close is the crash, the violation, the abuse; too far and the system falls apart, there's no interest, no attachment, little mutual reciprocity or connection.

## The invisible line

Boundaries are that invisible line which we've often felt if, for instance, someone we don't know stands too close. On a physical level we can feel like we want to step back to give us more room. On a mental level, when someone judges us and says something personal 'ooh what a lot of spots you have', or 'you've put on weight' this can be 'overstepping the mark' of our boundaries. Think of the question, 'what do you think you are doing?' and the invasive qualities and impact that can have on us.

Boundaries are a very important aspect of our self-care and learning more about these interpersonal boundaries can give us some perspective and understanding of how we relate and interact with the world. Drawing the lines can make the difference between energetic nourishment and depletion, protection from others who take from us and maybe even to protect others if we are 'taking energy' from them without having realised that. We are human and not perfect and if we don't know or realise, because we were never taught about boundaries, then we may have overstepped the mark ourselves. Society has a dysfunctional perspective on boundaries, encouraging codependent relationships for instance. Reading a few books about them could make a difference to many areas of your life, particularly if you aren't that assertive.

## Enmeshment

One of the difficulties that we may have in understanding self-care is when other people are seen as being extensions of ourselves, rather than separate. Love songs often portray this and the phrase 'the other half', could well be changed to the 'other whole'. The royal 'we', e.g. 'we like that don't we', as mother may say about daughter, can demonstrate where boundaries are blurred and ill-defined. The daughter may well be rendered speechless and overpowered by her mother and unable to say, 'no, actually I don't'. This blurring of the boundaries is called enmeshment. It frequently happens in codependent relationships or friendships, where couples are very close. Similarity may be a feature or a necessity, rather than acceptance of healthy differences or interdependent ways of being.

# Compulsion to help

This may well go hand in hand with enmeshment. The wounded healer is someone who is compelled to want to heal others because they have felt such sorrow or trauma in their life, they don't want anyone else to feel like that, so try to resolve their wounds by 'healing' others. Sometimes this is to avoid looking at their own wounds; it's a great distraction but can cause dysfunction within the therapeutic relationship.

A co-dependent caretaker, is someone who is over-identified in the role of therapist. They don't switch off when they go home. They are often a rescuer and very much enjoy helping others. They may feel a (burning!) compulsion to help others when they see someone is struggling. Instead of taking a step back and seeing if that person can do it by themselves, and grow from their own experience of pushing through that, someone who has this compulsion may feel very guilty (see toxic guilt), mean and selfish if they don't 'do' for the other person. It is likely that this could be because by sparing others their pain, they don't have to feel their own unresolved pain within.

The key is to look to resolve our own pain through SC. That key gives us the freedom from compulsion, it is the gateway to growth not just for us but for others too. When we realise this, and do our own SC healing work, we can hold a true genuine space for others to grow as we fully allow them to just be, as they are, in a non-judgemental space.

# Victim, rescuer, persecutor

This dynamic, known as the Karpman triangle, is initiated when someone sends out a plea for help and it is a chronic or dysfunctional way of relating. The need for help may be hinted at rather than asked for outright, for instance 'I haven't got anyone to feed the rabbit', instead of 'can you feed the rabbit please? I'm going away'. Those of us who like to help and to be needed will then quite happily help to rescue the situation; after all, there maybe a payoff for us too (spending time with the lovely rabbit!) However, over time or too frequently, this dynamic can set up a vicious circle, especially if the person is doing this intentionally. They may be sending out hooks for help because they don't take responsibility for themselves. In this scenario they are not doing anything to help themselves i.e. organising someone to feed the rabbit, before they say yes to plans to go away.

Some people may enjoy being taken care of in this way. They like being rescued as it can absolve them of responsibility and in genuine cases, of course, it's a relief to have help. Sometimes it's nice to be rescued! Others, however, may find their boundary (space) feels trodden on or violated as they have a wider boundary and would prefer to do things themselves. They may even complain that the person is 'fussing' or 'interfering'. They may snap at the rescuer and by doing so they persecute. They have gone from being a 'victim' to being the 'persecutor', who then becomes the victim. Immediately they may feel sorry for snapping at them and try then to soothe them and rescue them.

This dynamic can go round and round in circles, sometimes one partner or friend is the rescuer and other times the victim. If the roles are fairly constant, the 'rescuer' may over time start to find the requests for help depleting, especially when the 'victim' isn't doing anything to help themselves. Feelings of annoyance and frustration kick in and can become 'persecutory'. We may start to feel or get a gut instinct that something isn't quite right, we may feel a little bit manipulated but battle internally with the part of us that feels sorry for them and makes excuses for them.

This was a wake-up call that I had when I realised that I was struggling with anxiety, depression and going out of the house. I was feeling depleted and overly saying yes to people when they were happily going about their daily lives. I took stock and thought, hang on this is out of balance, I began to take more responsibility for saying no. It wasn't easy, as I so automatically said yes to helping people without even thinking. I still can fall into this trap from time to time. It's can be a habitual automatic dynamic, but self-awareness, and SC can really help change this so that we can make more mindful choices as to whether we say yes or no.

The circle needs to be broken, either by suggesting that the 'victim' might need professional help for whatever they are struggling with, and some sort of intervention if necessary and there are services for that. Someone who is frequently complaining about the same problem in their life, but doing nothing about it can be draining to be around. I hold my hands up to this one too. I've worn all the t-shirts and this is often the case if we are able to be honest with ourselves, as with the circle we take on all the roles.

The key is taking responsibility and action. This is done by taking a step back, putting a boundary in place which says 'time to take responsibility for me here'. Perhaps both parties need to seek professional advice such as therapy, instead of trying to rescue each other. We are not our partner's or friend's therapist, this again is a blurring of the boundaries which may have evolved from dynamics in childhood.

# And so the therapist is born

The caretaking dynamic can be born of early relationships, sometimes what is known as 'parentification' where the roles are reversed and the parent has assumed the child role in the relationship. A common scenario is when a mother or father says 'you make me angry', they have given the child the power to determine their emotions, rather than as an adult saying 'I feel angry with you' (but I can handle my emotions myself, you aren't responsible for me). Another common example is if responsibility falls on the young male children in the family, if the father leaves, to be head of the family - 'you're the man of the house' now.

Similarly expressions such as 'don't cry or you'll make me cry' suggests that the child becomes caretaker of the adult's emotions. Realising that Mum can't cope with her own emotions, they have to guard and suppress their own so not to upset her. The hurt and tears that they may be feeling come second to the mother's, they become less important and also learn in the process how to put themselves aside. Emotions become repressed and the child assumes what is an adult role. Children who are seen to be 'little adults', mature for their age or precocious may have been raised with this dynamic. I think many counsellors and therapists may have been 'created' this way. They have been 'trained' from a young age to put themselves aside and to listen to others. They learn to sacrifice themselves and feel overly responsible for others in the process. It becomes a very natural, normal chronic dysfunctional dynamic. With seemingly the best of intentions.

# The road to hell

However that doesn't help you if you are compelled to give at a cost to yourself, because the worst case scenario of that is burnout. This leads to frustration, irritation, annoyance, fatigue, depression and anxiety. And that is the shadow side to the care industry and where I believe that abuse can begin to happen if we do not pay more attention to self-care, when often good intentions were the premise.

When people are tired and irritable, they care less; they take less care - and there's something in that turn of phrase. Undoubtedly it would benefit those in that position to take more care for themselves. Why do we think we are different to the phone or car in the need for maintenance? I cannot reiterate this enough, for the flow of life, for vitality to be felt we must receive as well as give otherwise there is something out of balance and something has to give. Sometimes this is us.

# TheRapist / therapeutic vampirism

This may shock you and perhaps it needs to, to help some of us have the wake up call before its too late! The shadow side, or the flip side to the therapist is theRapist.

This is the dark side of the work that we do. You may be shrinking and feeling horror at this suggestion and it is important to take note. I'm not talking about physical rape, although that sadly can also happen, but I am talking about energetic rape.

Have you ever felt torn off a strip, violated, put down? Sometimes we take power from others in different ways in order to recharge ourselves. Snidey comments, little put downs, jokes which really aren't funny and little digs are all power snatches. These are an attempt to recharge and make those who do this feel better about themselves. One-upmanship, a competitive nature and superior feeling are all ways of gaining energy or power from others. Trying to control them, telling them what to do because 'we know best', giving unsolicited advice, they can all be forms of energetic or mental rape.

Unfortunately, in my experience, this 'I know best' form of mental rape happens quite frequently in spiritual circles, particularly mind body spirit fairs. This is a form of spiritual abuse. There are many wounded healers on this path who are seeking power and their voice to be heard. I have the t-shirt for that one too, that I have worn and still don, with aspirations not to! By it's very nature of 'oneness', spirituality is unboundaried. 'We are all one', 'we are all connected', but in the wrong hands this is taken to mean that boundaries are ignored (and quite often misunderstood) and everyone is fair game. What is often thought to be OK in these circles is that 'if I perceive I'm being given psychic information, I'm going to tell you', whether you want to know or not. A respectful boundary would be to ask if the person is interested in hearing something that you feel you may be picking up, if you really need to say something at all. Oftentimes it can be self-serving.

I often tell this story when I teach psychic development about something that unfolded early in my development. Although I wouldn't intend to read someone without their permission, one Christmas I thought about choosing a few angel cards, which were positive and thought this would be nice for people to include in their Christmas cards. However, they hadn't asked for them and I saw in one friends card, with horror, a scenario that she would be splitting with her partner. That was the first and last time I did that. I didn't tell her as she hadn't asked, but this is what I mean by the road to hell is paved with good intentions. We may feel like we are doing the 'right' thing for people.

I've seen, felt this and been on the receiving end of many of these things from well-meaning therapists and caregivers myself, as well as those who give very forceful unsolicited advice - 'what you need to do is…'. It arises from a lack of self-awareness that none of us are immune to either. We all can do things without being aware and this is why as a therapist, I repeatedly convey the importance of personal development, so that we can be a clean clear channel for others. This comes first and foremost. From my point of view I do not want to do another any harm and would be very sad to think that in the course of my work I had hurt someone out of my own need for power.

## Power issues

A very big part of self-care is to look at our power issues and ways in which the ego can trap us into thinking that we can override another's boundaries. The ego is a very dicey player, it isn't all about 'I'm great at this, aren't I fab, with my large head?'. It can be about the fear that we aren't good enough so have to compensate or about thinking that others are better than we are and feeling jealous and wanting to quash them, rather than remembering our uniqueness. It has a function in trying to keep us safe and protected in its own way; but it also forms defences that sometimes we may have outgrown.

Realising that I am human and will likely make mistakes, I set an intention and prayer years ago to God in regard to my therapeutic work and readings, to ask that 'were I ever to do something out of my awareness...' (because with the best will in the world we are human, we have foibles, irritations and off days)', that would harm another, please put an obstacle in my path'.

I think many of us have had treatments from other therapists who have ended up over-talking about their problems during treatments. Some of the time I don't mind a little of this because as fellow therapists we can benefit from the exchange, however when I am silent during the treatment and the therapist then breaks the silence, repeatedly and talks about what's going on in their life, they are taking energy. From an energy perspective, that's dire and this is the dark side of the therapist. I will hold my hand up, I've done it myself and had to rein myself in, it's usually a call that we need to take it to therapy. I have worn many t-shirts and made and will probably still make mistakes and it is about learning from them.

Self-disclosure during therapy sessions may sometimes be appropriate, because it maybe helpful for the client to understand that they are not alone in experiencing something and it happens to others too; however, if we need to do it or feel compelled to it, that's a red flag for self-care help. It is worth checking in with the client if they feel it is helpful, otherwise we maybe taking our self-care too far if it becomes all about ME! Bringing us back to boundaries, this really is a boundary violation, we are invading the clients space and stealing their time with us.

# Professional limitations

We need to know our professional limitations are both a boundary and self-care. Knowing what we can handle and what we can't and referring on to others where possible helps to keep the client safe. If someone comes to me with a sports injury, I would refer them on to another for sports massage. When a client's back isn't getting better after a few treatments, I will suggest they see an osteopath or if they seem emotional or stressed perhaps a counsellor. If we try too hard, to take responsibility for another that needs something else, we may end up damaging them, God forbid, or being drained. We can't save the world, sometimes a client would be better off with another therapist who has different skills to help them. It's not defeat, it's not failure, it's not about you and it can actually generate energy because it will empower the client and yourself knowing that you are doing the best for them.

# Professional boundaries

And on that note it brings me fluttering back to that idea that the road to hell is paved with good intentions and the story of the caterpillar and the butterfly, from the Healer Heal Thyself chapter. I'm not a great believer in hell as a place, but think it can certainly be felt here on earth and perhaps it is up to us to create our heaven!

When we are givers and when we enjoy taking care of others and helping them with genuine empathy, it can be very hard to see someone struggling. With empathy, we walk in the other's shoes, so often bring the scenario back to ourselves, imagining how it would feel. That can be tough going and heart rending. The depths of pain can crack our heart open, not literally but on an energetic basis. This can enable us to hear with deep empathy. It can help us to hold that space to allow another to feel their own pain so that they can accept it to let it go. If I hadn't allowed myself to go to my own depths, I couldn't allow another, because effectively I'd be trying to rescue them so I wouldn't have to feel MY pain. It is our pain that we are feeling, our unresolved pain when we try to rescue or save another.

You may be thinking that it is cruel to let someone go through that. I love the adage from the angels that they will not give us help unless we ask for it or it is life-saving. The step that I took back from my previous relationship, I knew would break my ex partners heart. I also knew that if we stayed together she would not grow. It was incredibly tough, but she has bloomed. Both of us have grown by not staying together.

When we have taken responsibility for ourselves and participated in our own healing and therapeutic journey, realised and grown from it, we can then learn to not jump in. So fighting that compulsion to do so and remembering that we cannot save the world, or the butterflies, can also mean that we go into energy conservation mode and allow those boundaries to be as they are. However, we all have blind spots. It can take many years to change old habits which do die hard, to become more aware and conscious of where we may get drawn in. It then brings in the N word.

## Saying no. Full stop.

This is a boundary biggy. And such a huge component of self-care and possibly why anyone would be reading this sort of book in the first place. A shared difficulty for all. 'No' means that I am valuing myself more than you. Crumbs! What's that all about? That I might actually have self-worth? That I could put myself first when I've been down the list for so long? Whoa!

I'm joking and being light-hearted but the truth of this is tragically sad, that we have so little self-regard or self-respect that many of us find it a hugely difficult thing to say no. When someone asked me to do something, as I have said, 'yes' fell out of my mouth automatically, I didn't even stop to think, no wasn't an option. That was how I'd been programmed and raised. I thought it was my job or role to be there at the beck and call of others, to do as they asked. The most tragic of this is that I didn't fully understand that I could say no to sex. Somewhere in the background of the tragedy was the voice that told me 'not to exaggerate', 'not to make a fuss', the ones that said when I was bullied at school that 'sticks and stones can break your bones but words can never hurt me', and the same one that said when living with a psychopath who violently smashed the house up, 'everyone has arguments'. Had a mirror been there for me - like many others - that said, 'this is not acceptable behaviour,' I probably might not be doing the job that I do.

Because, like others who travel the oft difficult path of the therapist, we have a history of it being the norm for our boundaries to be violated. This in part is because boundaries weren't understood. Psychological education is really advancing now and we have suffered more from ignorance perhaps than wrong intention. As a consequence many of us, like myself, have literally had to find our true selves and rebuild an identity. I had none, it had been over-ridden by the wounded wants and needs of others. So I fully appreciate how difficult it can be to say no, it's like creating a new person. And there are occasional times when I still do say yes when perhaps I'd like to say no. This is why it is so important to look to what our wants and needs are, that we do matter, we do count, and in that we begin to build a sense of self worth, contained within boundaries that protect us from these kind of tragic experiences. We need to rekindle the flame and the light that fills us again.

## Unboundarified niceness

Not so long back I went to a spiritual evening. I had fancied finding out more about a particular group, who I'd often encountered when I was younger, and who always seemed happy. Seeing an advertisement I went along and had a very enjoyable evening. The group leaders were welcoming and explained various aspects of the beliefs and it culminated in a delicious vegan supper. With all good intentions, many of the devotees came to chat and find out more about me, one couple wanted to buy me a book, a few others to give me their phone numbers. There were suggestions with others that we meet up, for me to phone another devotee when she'd had no idea who I was: 'here's their number'.

I began to feel a little bit overwhelmed, with all good intentions. Had I not been where I'm at now, I can see I would have ended up in some very sticky situations as I have in the past when I'd just jumped into friendships taking people at face value. I'd say to myself 'oh they're nice because they are friendly and paying me attention', 'they're good people because they are spiritual' and jump right in. I'd regretted it in the past because I'd get too involved, too soon, without taking time to get to know whether people are right for me or not. Through SC I meet many more of my own needs for attention; I pay heed and attention to myself. I made my excuses and didn't feel the need to contact them again, there wasn't any guilt, just a very good demonstration of how unboundaried spirituality with the best of intentions can be, which isn't necessarily always a 'good' thing.

# Shut-up!

Self-care may also be about realising that we do not need to divulge so much information, especially so soon in a relationship or friendship. The reason why I call this section shut up, is because when we are too open, we are literally leaving ourselves vulnerable not only mentally but spiritually too. Those who's intentions aren't so kind can latch on to us, hook us in and drain us. They take power and learning not to open up to people who cannot appropriately handle that power can be trial and error, or error and error as I have found! There is something to be said for conserving your own energy and not letting it drain out of you. If you yourself are very talkative, you may benefit from going to counselling or some other therapist such as Reiki. With the tongue in cheek section title, shutting up may actually be about allowing ourselves or learning how to shut the door, to close down, so that we don't remain so open to certain others.

# Emotional blackmail

The tactic of emotional blackmail effectively gets us to relinquish our space so someone can invade it and take from us. It can be overwhelming or uncomfortable when people intrude upon us and take something from us that they need and we may not feel we have enough of. It is a form of theft! When we begin to realise the tactics that others employ to get their needs met we may notice how our feelings are triggered. This can be a sign that something is going on.

Sometimes when behaviours are manipulative and we begin to see through that intentional manipulation we can feel angry and rightly so. We may also feel used, silly, naive. Anger may be an uncomfortable emotion for us to feel, but please remember anger can be a sign that our boundaries have been violated. It can also be a release of energy that has been freed which can then be redirected into assertion! When we recognise that we have been manipulated we may then be more able to say No to reinforce, maintain and protect our boundaries from others! Go and make your own energy please!

'No.' is a complete sentence. We do not need to justify or explain ourselves if that person is pushy. If we do, it is likely that we will be getting drawn in by someone who is challenging us and trying to push the boundary and get us to change our mind. 'No.' as a complete sentence forms a boundary.

Recognising these things can take years. We all have our blind spots. Today mine was a kitten. Of course I wanted to keep an eye on it when it's new owner was going out! This is the sort of stuff where there's a lovely pay off for us too and a conscious choice to help another because we have extra energy and we aren't too tired or drained too. Asking ourselves what is the cost to me and am I OK with this before we proceed can help us to mindfully decide if we have the available energy. That is self-care and energy conservation.

So to wrap up this chapter with a closing boundary, we've looked at how those invisible lines called boundaries are the space around us which protects us and allows us to be ourselves. These 'fences' can become invaded, depleted, entwined or enmeshed with others. We may end up giving away too much of ourselves, we may by getting caught up in the victim, rescuer, persecutor cycle and need professional help and some of this might be because of our upbringing and society's dysfunctional teaching, how skewed our sense of responsibility is. These are all huge topics in themselves which I haven't been able to include all of the facets of because they are books in themselves. Nevertheless, there are pointers for you to go away and look into further. I recommend Anne Katherine's book 'Where you end and I begin' for more information if this is something that interests you further.

# Chapter Ten

## Take Action!

### Take action - just do it

This is the shortest section in the book - for the very reason that we often over-think our self-care and don't get on and do it!

How often do we promise ourselves that we will take better care of ourselves, then put off making the phone call to book in with a counsellor, or make an appointment to have our feet attended to? Or need to phone the hairdresser, or will sit down in a minute just after I've done this or this and this, or we will start meditating tomorrow…

When we take action, we generate energy. Over-thinking can often get in the way of taking action, we can put ourselves off before we even begin. I remember trying to get over my dental phobia. Every time I went to the dentist and had any work done, especially a filling, I fainted and had a seizure. This had happened so many times that it was off-putting and impractical, so I hadn't summoned enough courage to go for a while. When I was teaching a Reiki 2 group I decided during the section on asking for healing for ourselves, that I always participate in too, that I would ask for help with my dental phobia.

# Being open to help

Within the next few days I was coming out of the local supermarket. Usually I would walk straight to the car with my bags and then go diagonally across the car park to the pet shop. This time my intuition firmly directed me to walk straight to the pet shop with my bags. After a moment, I did so and noticed as I walked past the dentist that they were taking on NHS patients. 'Go in', urged my intuition. Meekly, I did so. I signed up and made an appointment. 'Put it out of your mind', said my intuition. When the date came for my appointment, for the first time in years I went by myself. I purposefully stayed in the moment and managed to do it, like at last I had a screen that was filtering out those fearful thoughts that can crowd in on us when we are scared. I realised I had to decide whether I liked the dentist and 'let him in'; I did like him and therein followed a gradual progression to recovery from the dental phobia.

# Acting on your intuition

How often have you had an intuitive thought, not acted on it at the time, then it happened? 'You'll drop the cup' says our intuition, 'No you won't' you argue with yourself as you carry the cup, the laptop, the sellotape, the pen, the notepad. 'You'll manage' says the ego. Crash! down goes the cup. 'Told you you should have listened to your intuition', the ego berates! When our poor intuitive voices go unheard time after time, they begin to fade into the background, until we learn to listen to them and act on them. This not only generates more energy, but strengthens our intuition so that we begin to hear more and more of it.

## 10. Take Action

What do you need to do? What have you said that you will do? What can you do right now? Do it (remember the rule as long as it harms none - no murderous thoughts about wringing your ex's neck are allowed to be acted upon!). But seriously, as you do what you have been meaning to do for a while, pay attention to yourself, notice how you feel and remember that feeling.

# Chapter Eleven

## Trust the Journey

Trusting in the journey and that things often do work out can be a relief to realise. Letting go and surrendering to the Powers that Be instead of feeling that we have to control everything can free up a lot of anxious tension.

Being self-employed is challenging, knowing that it is up to ourselves to bring in the money to pay the bills. In the early stages of working as a holistic therapist I was very fortunate that my partner then had a decent job and because I'd not been working, everything else that I made was a plus for us, as long as I covered my therapy room rent. The first time I earnt £5 via a donation treatment, I felt like I'd won the lottery, as I had very little money! I remember thinking I might be able to afford treatments myself soon. It is said that it takes at least two years to build up clients and get a full diary. And it certainly did take a while. Like many people, I did envisage that there would be queues of people knocking my door down to get in, when I began renting my room at the centre where I work. I served myself up a large piece of humble pie whilst I realised that was my ego talking, but I did find that there was enough. I'd felt that as long as my rent got paid I was to remain in business.

There have been, in the last ten years, only a couple of occasions when the money for the rent has literally come in at the eleventh hour. That's not to say it's been easy, being self-employed I don't get holiday pay or sick pay, so taking time off 'costs' money. I have often tentatively booked time off knowing that having no clients during that time means no income and also knowing that money even for the basics or to pay to go away has to come from somewhere. I began to learn to trust that there was a process happening where things did work out OK, but still I had some anxiety about taking time off. When my then partner was made redundant there was an added pressure on us and I went into worry mode again and stayed there for a good few years.

However, in time I began to settle the anxiety. I entered a deeper level of trust, as over and over again things worked out, if the diary was quieter and certain bills needed to be paid, someone might buy a gift voucher. I would no longer frantically panic when my diary was quiet and it has become an interesting game of observing how the powers that be are going to provide. I tune in to find out my part of the greater plan and show up to do my job with integrity.

The Powers that Be undoubtedly plan my diary for me, I realised this very early on. There is a bigger picture going on, an energy that knows when I may need more time to clean my therapy room, or do admin or have time for myself. Now I tend to think 'hmm what I am going to be doing?' in that quiet slot, rather than always trying to fill it. Sometimes it might that someone wants a last minute appointment, or 'God slot' as I sometimes call it! I may have ideas and things I might like to do, such as course work, but I tune in and listen for advice from the best spiritual PA! It usually works out. Cancellations can sometimes be fortuitous for others as it can create a space for someone in need and if that happens the person who has cancelled doesn't get charged a cancellation fee.

From a self-care perspective, trust in this amazing process, stops me from worrying. I used to wake up nearly every morning worrying. I knew realistically that worry is fear of the future and to stay in the moment, but I woke up with that energy. I needed to learn to just Let Go and Let God (please translate to your own Divine guidance if appropriate).

# Synchronicity

The degree of synchronicity that I experience in my daily life is very reassuring. This is where 'a coincidence' seems too great, for it not to be meaningful. These are my indicators and signposts, also my 'heart gladden-ers'. For example, just as I'm editing, two Jehovah's Witnesses knock on my door. I could ignore the door as I don't really have time to get into conversation (ie I'm remaining closed to what life is bringing me, by closing myself off, when I've asked for help with my book and my life).

I answer the door and there are two ladies, they are radiating heartfelt smiles, which is nice to see. I explain that I am busy and they ask if they can leave me with a leaflet, which I'm happy to have. Despite differing beliefs, I appreciate that God gets a message across in whatever way! There are many paths up the same mountain. On the leaflet the message tells me that 'with God all things are possible', I feel supported as I've asked for help with the book. I sit in gratitude. So asking for support and the subsequent unfolding of these synchronistic events indicate when I am in the flow of life. I am connected to something greater which helps to guide and navigate me through life and the decisions. Ultimately the decisions are mine, I am responsible for the choices that I make.

# Change

When we embark on lifestyle changes, it can be scary and it can also scare those around us. To accommodate the changes that we make, others may also have to adapt. As we change they are either forced to change themselves in some way or other or in response or make the decision not to and the friendship or relationship ends. This is not only growth, or moving out of place where we have been stuck, it stirs things up and can be very uncomfortable. A simple example may be that we decide that we aren't going to get home at 5pm on a Wednesday night but instead go to yoga on the way home from work. The knock-on affect on other family members around meal times may cause them to have to take more responsibility, to protest and it may seem quite a battle.

It's said that the only certainty in life is that things change. The world is in a constant state of flux. It goes back to the concept of Impermanence and understanding that can also help us to embrace changes - 'feel the fear and do it anyway!' Courage isn't absence of fear. It is quite normal to be nervous about change.

As you have been reading this book, you may find that you have to take an honest look at your lifestyle and make some changes which at first you may find hard. You may be in denial about certain things. Change may not be immediate or a magic wand, making small changes gradually can still work over time and it is often unrealistic to expect too much too soon.

Making a variety of changes to your lifestyle will invariably be more effective than making just one change and waiting for miraculous results, however you may not know then whether it's an individual factor that has worked or several factors combined! Holistic therapies take into account the whole person, who is often governed and effected by a number of factors – it may not just be one thing that causes the imbalance. Multiple factors may play a part such as diet and exercise along with mental and emotional stressors, and maybe even spiritual factors too. Addressing as many of these factors as possible, not just one at a time, may help to get your body back into balance.

In part II of the book we look at Balms to Self-Care which, with your new found freedom from all the obstacles that you've put in the way of your self-care in the past (I say this tongue in cheek, it is ongoing please remember), will provide examples that can empower you to put self-care into practise.

# Part II

## How We Can Self-Care

# Chapter Twelve

## Complementary Therapies & Supervision

### Holistic & Complementary Therapies

This is my go-to form of self-care. I have weekly treatments and adore them, so I am a good advertisement for my own job! I only offer the treatments that have helped me. My first experience of holistic therapies was when my sister paid for me to have an aromatherapy massage. I was very nervous, as I was depressed and highly anxious. I worried about getting undressed too and felt self-conscious. After the massage, I felt almost drunk, I was so relaxed and had never felt that relaxed before in my life. I was glad my sister drove me home! Over the years I then tried others, such as homeopathy, Reiki, osteopathy, reflexology and so on, and have had quite profound experiences with many of them.

Regular - or even occasional - holistic therapies can help with our mental, emotional, spiritual and physical personal development and self-care. I think that they also help us to become better therapists as they are a form of continued professional development, as everyone works in a different way and from that we can learn much from colleagues or therapists. I also liken it to a good battery recharge and clearing, as we are getting a top up or boost from another therapist which we can then take back to our clients/families etc., so it benefits us all.

Givers are notoriously bad receivers so it can take some self re-training! I feel engagement and the 'allowing' of this is about letting another person into our space and that it helps me to be a better therapist than I would be without it, because of the benefits I get from that. It's like a support system, or team, behind me as I do for others, rather than feeling like I have to do it all by ourselves. I've also observed on numerous occasions how reluctant therapists can often be to pay for their own therapies, that there can often be blocks there to allowing it. Shrugging off treatments or counselling with other therapists or only doing the minimum requirements for self-care, rather than it being the norm can not only lead to burnout, but poor practise and ethics.

The benefits of therapeutic touch, in my experience, can be restorative. For those who grew up with few hugs and little physical and emotional support, regular therapies I feel can help restore that balance. I see this also with clients who have experienced difficult childhoods, or trauma as adults, as treatments are so effective at soothing the nervous system. I think that they retrain or teach the body how to relax. Many of us may have not experienced such a deep sense of relaxation before.

## Is it the placebo effect?

It may help if we have belief in something and perhaps that can be a factor. However, having seen how my cat Poppy responded to homeopathy, how my friend's horse responded to the herb turmeric (and the other went loopy!) and just recently how our cat Pepper responded to homeopathy. It highlights that something else is going on, as animals aren't susceptible to placebo. They don't know what they've been given (I would also say here that by law in the UK, treatments for animals must be administered by a qualified vet. I'd also add as an aromatherapist, that I would be very careful about using essential oils with animals, they are chemicals and animals can have some strong negative reactions to them). I was so ill, and struggling to get through each day, that ultimately I came to the conclusion, like many people that suffer from chronic illness, that I didn't give a flying fig about whether it was placebo or not anyway if it worked and helped to alleviate my suffering. I often still have one foot in sceptic; we really don't know how a lot of this works, there isn't much scientific evidence (and I'm sceptical about that too as I think there are too many variables in life to say for sure). I still find that I can't quite fully believe that certain therapies work in the way that they do, crystal therapy for instance, but I know I've had profound experiences with crystals, that they do work for me. I think the placebo argument can also be used as obstacle by people who don't want to take responsibility for their own health, by looking at finding other things that will help them. Plus fear, because if it were to work what would change? My whole life did, for the better!

## Frequency

Because we are all different, because we don't know exactly how some of these things work (but have some good theories and possibilities) I will say to clients who come, no promises no guarantees that they will work. If you don't feel at least relaxed during the treatment, try something else. If you feel relaxed and benefit in other way like your aches and pains subside, great - it may be an indication that the treatment will work for you. I suggest they tune into their body and ask it if they need more treatments. A course of treatments, particularly if someone has been chronically ill for a long time, will help to get the ball rolling, then when you start to feel better, taper the regularity out so instead of coming weekly, you come fortnight or three weekly.

# Ethical therapists

An important aspect of your self-care is to find yourself an ethical therapist, one who is perhaps recommended, who is a member of a professional body and importantly that you feel comfortable with. You will have a consultation which helps the practitioner to understand more about your medical condition, so that they can best care for you.

Clients can feel in a vulnerable position lying on a therapy bed, so we need to create that safe space and treat them with dignity whilst undressing and kept covered during the treatment when that area is not being worked on. For those who are nervous or sensitive, treatments can be taken step by step, so that they can fully relax and know that they are in control of the treatment at all times. Ethical therapists won't encourage you to spend beyond your means. Sadly, I have heard of a practitioner encouraging people to overspend and take a loan out, to have twice weekly treatments that they were recommended.

## Aromatherapy massage

Aromatherapy is the therapeutic use of essential oils, which may benefit the health of mind, body and spirit. Essential oils all have different therapeutic properties, a good example which many of us have experienced is the decongestant properties of eucalyptus. Other oils may be prized for their anti-depressant properties or their analgesic (painkilling) properties, for example, and most oils have more than one therapeutic use. As Hippocrates said, "The way to health is to have an aromatic bath and a scented massage every day", lovely! The practitioner will select essential oils according to your personal preferences as well as the health conditions that you would like to address. These oils are then used for your massage.

**The potential benefits of aromatherapy massage**
- Stimulates circulation
- Stress relief
- Detoxification & lymph drainage
- Emotional & mental benefits
- Touch/contact benefits
- Stimulates immune system & increases resistance to disease
- Allergy relief
- Removal of lactic acid
- Promoting healthier skin

# Reflexology

Reflexology is a treatment which applies pressure to specific parts of the feet or hands in order to stimulate the body's own ability to heal itself. An image of the body is said to be reflected in the feet, so when pressure is applied to certain areas, this can help the parts of the body that the point corresponds to e.g. the edge of the foot corresponds with the spine and can be focused on if someone is suffering from a bad back. Reflexology can benefit physical conditions as well as mental and emotional ones. Often people who complain that their feet are 'too tickly' find that the pressure that is used during a reflexology treatment is surprisingly comfortable for them, and not tickly, but relaxing. Lotion, oil or talc is used on the feet. Most people find reflexology to be a relaxing treatment; similar to having the feet massaged.

One theory of how Reflexology works is based on energy channels, or zones, within the body. The aim of a treatment is to bring the energy of the body back into a state of balance. There are thought to be ten zones, or channels, which are linked from the hands and feet to other parts of the body, such as the liver or the neck. By stimulating the reflexes or acupressure points on the feet, energy is stimulated to help the body to heal itself. Each part of the hand or foot is linked to a specific part of the body, for example the eyes or the spine and these body part are shown on reflexology 'maps', which are pictures of the feet. When these points are stimulated in the corresponding body the energy can once again flow freely. Energy blockages are thought to manifest in the feet or hands as 'crystals' which feel 'crunchy', or tender. As the crystals are broken down by massage the body may then begin to heal itself and health and well-being may be restored. Some conditions may benefit quickly from reflexology treatments, other chronic conditions may take a course of treatments.

*"The foolish man seeks happiness in the distance; the wise grows it under his feet."* James Oppenheim

**What may reflexology help with?**
- Insomnia
- Back & neck pain
- Aches and pains
- Water retention
- Mental & emotional problems
- Menstrual & menopausal problems
- Supporting IVF treatment
- Supporting body & aiding detoxification during smoking cessation
- Detoxification
- Digestive problems/constipation

Please remember no results are ever guaranteed, if it helps you to relax then that's a plus in itself. One frequent observation over the years of doing reflex treatments for people is that when people get off the bed they are surprised at how their bare feet feel as if they are walking on air cushioned soles!

# Reiki

Reiki (pronounced ray-key) is an ancient Japanese technique which involves a practitioner channeling energy and directing it to people or animals. Reiki has no association with any religion or faith and can be received by anyone who would like to experience this energy. It is a safe treatment; the person will only get what they can handle or need. Reiki is suitable for adults, elderly people, children and babies. A full treatment lasts 1 hour. The client remains fully clothed during the treatment. Reiki can be received lying down or sitting in a chair. The practitioner will place their hands on, or above, the client's body.

The sensation's experienced as the Reiki energy is received can range from intense heat, chills, cold, tingling, pressure and some people see colours. For most people, receiving Reiki is a deeply relaxing experience which promotes a feeling of well-being and peace. For others it can be an opportunity for emotional release, a chance to talk, or they may simply fall asleep.

### What conditions may Reiki help with?

Reiki may help to cleanse the body of toxins, relieve pain, soothe shock, or calm the mind. Everyone's experience and their reaction to Reiki is different and no two treatments per person will be the same. There are many conditions which may benefit from Reiki, a few of which are:

- Stress
- Chronic pain and general aches and pains
- Mental health problems
- Nervous system disorders
- Digestive problems
- Spiritual crisis
- Bereavement
- Sleep problems and disorders
- Trauma and shock

Reiki works alongside medical treatments and other complementary therapies.

## Holistic facials

The beauty of facials is that they aren't just for beauty! There are different types of facials, and if you select a facial type such as a holistic facial there can be quite a lot of massage. For those who hold tension in their face, and jaw, a facial can be a great way to work on those areas. Using essential oils that are tailored to your skin type and according to your preferences, a facial is a very relaxing way to treat your skin and to help ease muscle tension in the face, head and scalp which is particularly relaxing if you are stressed. It may help to improve your skin's complexion due to the cleansing effects of the products used which are selected according to your skin type. A facial massage increases circulation and stimulates the skin. After a facial many people notice that their skin glows! Some people experience outbreaks of spots as toxins are released from the skin, but with regular treatments the skin can clear.

**The potential benefits of a facial**

- Stress and facial tension relief
- Healthier skin
- Stimulates circulation
- Detoxification & lymph drainage
- Emotional & mental benefits
- Touch/contact benefits
- Relief of tension in jaw, face and scalp
- Sinus drainage

It's important to remember that what we eat has a huge bearing on the skin so attention to diet and nutrition may also be helpful.

# Indian Head Massage

Indian Head Massage, sometimes known as Champissage, originated from the Ayurvedic tradition in India. As a family practise, mothers would massage their children, and women would massage each other's hair for the benefits gained in relaxation and improved condition of the hair. It is a nurturing massage. Indian Head Massage has become a popular treatment and is suitable for the workplace, as the treatments last less than an hour. During the treatment the client has a choice of wearing a light top or t-shirt, with the massage done over the clothing, or they may prefer to remove their upper clothing (with a towel used to ensure modesty) and oils used directly on the back. The client stays seated upright in a low backed chair (or the therapist may ask the client if they would prefer to lie down on the therapy bed). The back, arms, neck, head and face areas are all massaged. The client also has the option of whether to have oil used in the hair, which may help to improve its condition.

If there is poor posture from sitting at the computer, reading or watching television, Indian Head Massage may help to ease tension in the neck. Some people tilt their head forward and the neck muscles then tense up to take the weight of the head. Massaging this area may help someone with a stiff neck to move their head about more freely. The shoulders are a common place for people to hold tension and people may stiffen there as a consequence. Massaging the shoulders may help to release anxiety or trapped energy and also increase mobility. Stiffness in the shoulders may cause imbalances throughout the body and have a knock on effect by restricting the ribs and therefore the breathing. It may also slow down the circulation and create headaches and impaired digestion. The head is covered in a fine layer of muscles which can tense up when anxious and lead to 'tension headaches' and migraines. Stress can appear as tightness around the mouth, forehead and eyebrows. During concentration our forehead and temples areas can become tight and congested which may limit blood flow, leading to eyestrain and tension headaches. Massage to the head may improve this flow.

**What conditions may Indian Head Massage help with?**
- Stress
- Muscle tension
- Detoxification
- Anxiety & depression
- Grief
- Increase circulation
- Tension headaches
- Improve hair condition
- Relieve eye strain

# Spiritual energy therapy

This might be also known as spiritual healing, shamanic work or similar. It may help in instances where we have felt 'dumped' on and the practitioner can help to clear blocks or cords of energy from the past or present, sometimes known as extraction work.

Usually the practise will be with a therapist who asks their spirit helpers to assist in the treatment. Work may be done on the aura to help to heal holes and energy channelled to plug in and recharge the person. Crystals, smudging, drumming, singing bowls and chanting may also form part of the treatment. During this time, spirit helpers or guides may work with the soul to retrieve and return soul part that have left, due to shock or trauma. Sometimes entity removal may feature if a person feels like they have what is sometimes known as an attachment from someone who has passed, an entity from elsewhere, or someone who is still alive. As always, it is good to contemplate the symbolic elements of these things, such as feeling like there is an alien attachment maybe a reflection of a shadow aspect of ourselves that we haven't integrated within ourselves.

After these energy clearing treatments the onus is on the person to try to keep doors shut, but it might be that their self-awareness needs to come from elsewhere, so exploring other treatments, if they wish, may help. For example, I kept being asked to clear someone's house, but because she kept watching horror films and scaring herself silly, she was leaving the energetic door open, so there was little more I could do. She gained something from it, because it gave her attention from others who would enjoy the theatrics of her having a 'ghost'.

# Giving up the reasons for being ill

In 'Why People Don't Heal' by Caroline Myss, I remember how she discussed that when we are chronically ill, it can be that we are holding onto hidden benefits that keep us stuck in that place. I was rather shocked at that. What benefits did I get out of being ill? Well it meant primarily, on some levels, that I didn't have to take responsibility for myself. That was a bitter transformational pill to swallow. I realised that by staying on Disability Living Allowance, I was compounding my sickness mentality, it was reaffirming to me that I was ill. I never liked being on it, I was ashamed, even though I did need it, until I got to a certain point. I am not for one instant saying here that people shouldn't be on it. If I could go back to myself in time, I would tell myself that it was OK and I needed it and to rid myself of the shame. However, it came to a point where I really wanted to embrace full wellbeing, move on and let go of the past.

Unsurprisingly, things unfolded! I went with my partner at the time to see the jets landing at Rhosneiger in Anglesey. Out of the blue, a woman standing beside me launched right into telling me about how ill she had been. She told me how she had now recovered, but how she had made the decision to come off benefits because she had to make the decision to be well. I couldn't get a word in edge ways so she knew nothing of my journey! It was exactly what I had been contemplating. Thank God for that lady. It gave me the courage to keep my mindset focused on one of wellness, a reassurance that I was on track as I made a leap. As that wellness was building up in me through my work, I knew I have made the right decision but it was scary letting go, rather like *Jump* with my eyes closed!

I did go through a phase of questioning this, when I went through a blip a few years back, but again realised that I was still able to work and function, difficult as that was at times and with support of supervision, and other therapies I was grateful that I was now in a place where I was able to take more time off for self-care, yet still be able to support myself. That backwards step showed me how far I had come.

# Homeopathy

Homeopathy has unfortunately received a lot of bad press recently, but I saw my cat benefit and that was enough for me to try it too, when I then had a profound experience. Within twenty minutes of taking the remedy that had been prescribed I felt a surge of energy coming up from my chest as an outpouring of grief commenced. I cried noisily, like I'd never cried before, all the suppressed grief that I had inside shifted out of me. When I stopped crying, I slept and the next day I was filled with such an incredible sense of peace, very similar to what I'd experienced when I had a near death experience. I could barely talk, my voice was so slow, like I was drunk. I was so very relaxed. I now know that the deep relaxation and slowing of my speech due to the clearing of my energy through homeopathy had taken me to another layer or a new level of profound awakening.

Homeopathy is an energy medicine and contains very little of the original substance that it is obtained from, which makes it hard for people to believe or understand because they can't see it. Once the person has had a remedy, (which doesn't always work as profoundly or noticeably as that with everyone) the person should find that they gradually just begin to get better and better, so looking back over the past six months, there has been an improvement. It may be a bit up and down, or backwards and forwards but overall there are improvements. The homeopath may then select a different remedy, as you begin to make changes in your life which affect your way of being, or 'remedy picture'. They treat the whole person. Homeopathy works on a principle of treating like with like, similar but not the same as a vaccination. I could see in some ways how it worked for my cat in a physical way (she was jaundiced, which was then alleviated), but was sceptical how it could work for me in a mental and emotional level, but I could not argue with that response! I still had work to do and it is a journey, but for me that was a significant turning point and the crux of why I do what I do. I won't say too much more about homeopathy, as I'm not trained, but having a look at the Royal College of Homeopaths will give you some more information and find a local practitioner if you fancy trying it.

## Counselling & psychotherapy

A counsellor works alongside their client to reflect back to them the issues that they may be having, in order that they begin to find their answers. It is empowering, it's a great space to have a vent or an outlet or to sort out issues that might be running through your mind or interfering with your day to day functioning. A counsellor won't tell you what to do or give you advice. As a member of the BACP or UKCP in the UK, they will have supervision in order to make sure that they are functioning with awareness in their role. There are many different forms of counselling, I didn't do well with Cognitive Behaviour Therapy (CBT) years ago because it didn't allow intuition to be a facet of it (no evidence), however I took the seeds and years later was able to sow them when the soil was more sterile and I had a flow of energy, to nurture the seeds, in my watering can! I think unless the deeper work is done, CBT can be like a plaster on a wound and a bit like hypnotherapy, we can convince ourselves by retraining certain thoughts to a degree, but the wound can then morph into something else and rear its head elsewhere. A person centred counsellor works in a reflective way, an integrative counsellor uses a combination of approaches and formed the fundamentals for my training (I am not a fully trained counsellor) as did Gestalt which I love because it embraces the mind body and spirit. There are also psychologists who have varying viewpoints, and I particularly liked the psychodynamic approach and Kleinian (which works with projective identification), but to my 'acceptance' I have not found a Jungian psychotherapist locally to do shadow work with as that is another approach I find particularly helpful. The recent combination of mindfulness with CBT is also an interesting approach which I feel can work well, again if the deeper work has been done.

## Supervision

Although technically work, this is still a very important aspect of self-care, because it cares for us at work, which is where we can deplete the most. 'Do no harm' and a desire to work for the highest good are intentions which, as helping professionals, support workers or carers, we genuinely strive to fulfil and uphold within our relationship with clients and others. At the same time we are human and therapeutic relationships are complex to begin with, let alone when we also have our own issues to contend with, which we may or may not be aware of. What do we do when our buttons get pushed and we suddenly feel overwhelmed with the realisation that we do not feel as able, much as we would like to, to remain unconditionally loving, grounded and centred? That can be a wake-up call and swift jolt back to reality. We are human after all.

## 12. Complementary Therapies & Supervision

When we first qualify in our work, it can be a lonely place out there if we are self-employed. You may be lucky enough to be working with others, or your trainer might still be on hand at the end of the phone to answer questions, and this can be reassuring. However, asking others for their help and advice might not always be possible and this is where a supervisor comes in. It helps us to offload, process and recharge and reignite. It is a fuelling station! However, even if this were to be made an industry requirement, some would still shrug it off, often due to a complete lack of awareness, and thinking that 'I am sorted and OK, I don't need it' because they genuinely don't see the reason, with the best will in the world. However, that is where denial can be our undoing; as with many helping professions, continued professional and personal development and the willingness to do that keeps us growing and prevents us from getting stale, as well as, importantly, keeping our clients safe.

A supervisor is someone who you can connect with regularly, for an hour or so each month to offload, or plough through the questions that have come up for you in practise that might be concerning or just niggling you. Whatever you want to bring to supervision you bring to supervision - it might even be how your personal life is affecting your work life. The supervisor isn't there to judge you or tell you what to do, they are there to walk alongside you.

A good understanding of boundaries and the therapeutic relationship may not have been part of your training as a helping professional. I do see this lacking in the practise of many therapists, (even counsellors) who are actually good therapists otherwise but don't understand how those boundaries can be part of the therapeutic dynamic in themselves. It's something I have struggled with too and still do from time to time. There is commonly a gap here, for now, yet it is a vital part of holding a safe space for the client during their therapy in order to give them room to grow. Codes of ethics may offer a way forward for the therapist to understand working safely with a client, but even these may be open to (mis)interpretation. I think the difficulty comes in because we find ourselves in real-world situations which are just not black and white, some boundaries are obvious such as not having sexual relations with clients. But it is the grey areas which can lead to confusion for anyone who works in relationship with another.

With confusion we can give out mixed messages and the energy and safe space of the therapeutic process is disrupted or lost. At worst, unintentional damage of your client may occur. This is where supervision comes into its own. It is there to ensure the safely and wellbeing of your clients, and sometimes your own safety where you maybe vulnerable too. It aims to walk alongside you (rather than telling you) to help you to navigate through any issues which may colour your judgement. That might be through a need for more therapy yourself or perhaps recommendation for further training. Good supervision is there for your client and supports your personal development and growth as a helping professional too.

Supervision can provide reassurance and support for you where you may be in doubt of your own abilities or it may support your growth where it is valid and needed. It is a point of contact for you to check in with you, to make sure that you are professionally and responsibly up to scratch which is also a fundamental aspect of your own self-care.

# Chapter Thirteen

## Meditation and Mindfulness

I'm pleased that a self-care book nowadays would not be that if it didn't contain information or reference to meditation and mindfulness. There is good reason for many why it is valued so greatly amongst those who struggle with stress and burn-out, if we can get our 'heads' and hearts around it. Possible reasons why we may struggle with it I'll speak about below. Common misconceptions can be misleading about meditation, which, once we let go of, may help ease us in to this technique and way of being.

Meditation was and is a big part of my wellbeing jigsaw, it made a significant difference that helped me deepen my healing journey. I'd had counselling and although it had helped in some ways, I still remained mistrustful of myself and without what is called 'internal locus of control'. This is where we have the belief that it is within us to control our lives. We don't recognise or believe in our own personal power to influence or make changes in our life. Meditation and understanding more about Buddhism helped me to reconnect to my true inner nature and begin that process of trusting myself, that I could begin to make a difference to my own life. It handed me back the reins. It empowered me and helped me to begin to believe in myself.

To illustrate some of the concepts, I will share some of my experiences. Many years ago, when I was at rock bottom, I attended relaxation classes at a mental health day-hospital. Relaxation classes usually teach people a process whereby each muscle is tensed and relaxed in turn, working up from the feet to the head. The feelings of tension and relaxation are noted in order to compare the difference and release some of the tension. This was helpful in teaching me to be more aware of how my physical body felt and endeavouring to make certain changes in posture, such as dropping my shoulders when they were tense and unclenching my jaw. We'd then do a visualisation of a beach, a place where it was nice to be, which wasn't always easy! My mind would stray and think about other things, I'd have a few glimpses of a beach but wonder how I'd ever get there in reality anyway! I'd also listen to relaxing music CDs in an aid to calm myself. This was all a good stepping-stone to meditative practise, and laid some foundations, but not something I experienced huge benefits from.

Twenty years ago, again in a dark place, a medium called Sue Winter tentatively told me that she felt that some of my experiences were due to psychic imbalances. She was apprehensive about making things worse for me though but felt that developing could help. She explained to me how to meditate and I was off and I flew! This was rapidly accompanied by the inner realisation that I needed to become more grounded! It was amazing, why wasn't this available on the NHS or in schools?! Fortunately it wasn't too many years later that arrived in the form of Mindfulness. I embraced the meditative practise that Sue had taught me and then attended some Buddhist classes and then over the years Mindfulness ones as they became popular. As well as what Sue had taught me about focusing on the breath, I used a variety of guided meditations on CD. I also had a cassette tape of self-hypnosis. This helped me to make headway in gaining a deeper state of relaxation initially in an attempt to overcome my tension, anxiety and nervousness, in order to let myself be (a bit!).

Practise taught me, as experience is the best teacher. I watched, observed, allowed - and also resisted many times over the years, as I did find it too much, too opening. Then I'd get an inner nudge to go back to it and continued and wonder why I hadn't worked through it and how I'd missed it, as we do. I was, however, safe in the knowing and non-judgement that 'it was as it was' and my journey unfolded, as will yours and that's OK. Without any formal meditation teacher as a constant, I surmised that what I was doing seemed to be closest to Vipassana or insight meditation which I believe is the roots of, or in my understanding very similar to, mindfulness.

One of the common misconceptions about meditation is that we are supposed to 'empty' the mind. However, I found like (probably everyone in the beginning, if that isn't too much of a generalisation) that I couldn't empty my mind of thoughts. It is the nature of the mind, or the 'monkey mind'. I therefore intuited that just sitting and noticing what came in, not attaching to or judging the thoughts, just watching them and letting them go, worked for me. I was making progress in meditation and with my engagement to life. When thoughts repeatedly come in, if I was worrying about something, I felt that the thoughts were trying to get my attention, so I would sit with them in contemplation. This was a deeper layer of insight into my healing journey. I felt it was my subconscious trying to get my attention.

If I sat with the repetitive thoughts and allowed myself to feel the feelings behind or underneath those thoughts and just be with those thoughts or sensations, insights and understanding, or 'teachings' would occur. I began to make sense of my motivations and receive insights which would then later be confirmed by life or reading it in a book. My sense was that I was tapping into what came to me as being a 'great pool of consciousness'. This is Jung's idea of the collective conscious, sometimes called the Akashic records. In this place, this state of being, the answers seem to flow. This was also where grounding came in, as I also realised that my creativity had opened up to the extent that I was thinking in rhyme. I realised that this wasn't allowing me to function in a healthy way, so backed off from it. There is a saying 'after enlightenment, chop wood', i.e. get back to basics to ground.

I had also been smoking cannabis to see if it helped with my depression. At this point I realised that although it was helping with my creativity, it wasn't helping my mental health. I felt I was verging on psychosis as the combination of that, the meditation and other practises was opening me up too much. I realised that taking substances was relying on something outside of myself to give an easy access, and questioned was it really 'real' if I had to do that to achieve those states? I hadn't used it in that way for that purpose; that was a by-product of using it for depression. So I stopped smoking it, practised more grounding (feeling the earth beneath my feet getting out in nature) and got back to me.

## Present moment awareness

The beauty of meditative practise, that can then occur quite naturally, is that it tips over into daily life as we become more conscious and present generally. As we begin to live that consciousness and awareness in the moment, everything in our daily life can become a meditation, such as doing the ironing or washing up, just bringing our attention and focus back to what we are doing. We may then not always sit in seated meditation practise. There can be many other ways of working with it such as chanting whilst out running or a mindful walking meditation. This means being conscious of our footsteps and relaxing with physical sensations in the body, noticing and observing what is occurring for us as we walk, listening deeply to nature and noticing and *feeling* the birds singing.

I have struggled with disciplined seated practise over the years off and on, however I've still progressed. If something isn't working for you right now, find another way, ask your inner-tuition how you best proceed at that point in your journey of self-care (see the Looking Within section). Self-care isn't about pushing the river, but sometimes we may need to ask ourselves whether we need to do a little steering of the boat. It's knowing what to do for our highest good (or best interests) and being honest with ourselves in any given moment. As I said, I've had times when the tide has been out and my life has been void of meditation. My sense was there would come a point when it would benefit me to work through my resistance and steer the boat or take the reins back, but in that moment it was OK to not do that and push myself. I also often feel that I experience the difficulties with many aspects of spiritual practises and personal development, so that I can better empathise or convey any learnings I've had to others when I work with them!

## Struggles to practise

I have found that meditation (as well as yoga) can open me up too much and is not right for me at certain times, it opens my flood gates of inspiration! It can vary for us all and it is our decision whether we decide to work through or acknowledge our resistances. We may need a formal teacher to accompany us on that journey and guide us through or find other tools to help support us. When we begin to work with spiritual practises or techniques, it can often be the case that we have an instant aptitude for it. After this honeymoon period is when the work begins, and working through it and other obstacles and learning curves may be part of that as we deepen our practise and go through the levels as it were.

It might even involve going away, engaging with life and reality and getting grounded, bringing mindfulness into daily life. Accepting that process can bring forth layers of development too, maybe the 'guilt' for not doing this wonderful thing that previously we've found so helpful (and cultivation of acceptance for where we are at). It might be understanding the severity of what I call my 'inner Sergeant Major'. This is our ego mind telling us 'we should' or 'ought do this or that' and shaking it's metaphorical finger at us. That might be about working out how to give ourselves more compassion instead and trusting the process. At some point we may begin to cultivate self-discipline with our practise. Like any other experience, it is a unique, personal journey, but one which has over the years of the tide going in and out, has brought me enormous benefit.

I like the analogy that I was shown out running one day, of how the tide going out leaves all the pebbles on the beach, and how beautifully they can glisten as the water has enhanced their colouring. The tide going out also exposes the rubbish that is left behind too. We may need to do a litter pick, and get rid of that rubbish before the next tide comes in (there is then essentially more room on the beach!). Over time we may also notice the gifts that are left behind in the pebbles, that the essence of the water is still there, that we can see the sea still, and as we progress more and more, the sea goes out less and less far, so that we can still maintain a connection even when it recedes slightly.

# Buddhist philosophies

Understanding some of the Buddhist philosophies has helped my psychological health enormously, and was similar to what my inner-tuition was guiding me to do, some of which are often included in mindfulness. The key concepts that I worked on, were non-attachment, where I endeavour to 'not attach to an outcome'. This meant cultivating more acceptance of 'what will be will be'. I can have a loose idea of how I'd like things to unfold and what I'd like to achieve and will work towards that, but if it doesn't happen or I notice obstacles, so be it. I know now that something else will occur and I trust in the flow of life that will be ultimately be for my benefit. So, rather than clinging to 'what I want', I accept what happens in reality with greater moment awareness.

In the early days, I questioned does this law of non-attachment mean that I can't have relationships anymore? It didn't, it just meant the acceptance that life does come and go. The Law of Impermanence illustrates that only change is a constant. Otherwise, everything in life changes, our thoughts, our feelings, nature, people. We are all in a state of transition. By assuming that things will stay the same forever, we cling to the past. It's gone. Staying in the present embraces the ever changing flow and rhythm of life. And the present is where we find the gift of joy.

# The pendulum swings both ways

I realised that in my desire for happiness, I had attached to that happiness when I was in a happy place. 'I want to stay like this forever', I'd wish. However, wishing isn't reality and just like life and the state of impermanence, the tide goes out and it comes in again, as do emotions. They go up and down and the Middle Path and finding that felt important to me. I'd often hear the phrase inside my head, 'the pendulum swings both ways before it reaches a place of balance'. Not attaching to that happy high, allowed me to accept that life can sometimes be unpleasant and allowing myself to feel that and accept it, rather than resisting it, was liberating. Being present to ourselves allows us the experience of being with the full gamut of our emotions, rather than suppressing them and cutting them off. It is important that we have sufficient tools such as a resilient self-esteem to help support us through that process.

## Contra-actions to meditation

As I have expressed in my own experience, meditation by its nature is opening. It does bring up some difficult periods as painful emotions can surface. I suspect this is why my meditation practise has come and gone over the years, and why support from a professional such as a counsellor, psychologist, holistic therapist or skilled mediation or spiritual teacher may be fortifying as you go through that process. By fortifying I mean, reflecting back an attitude of non-judgement to you in order for you to practise that within yourself. It is often the self-compassion that we lack which makes these emergences of emotions, become emergencies or crisis points.

## Our potential energy - Kundalini or spiritual awakenings

We can experience a myriad of symptoms if our Kundalini energy rises. But what is Kundalini energy? This energy is our *potential* energy and we all have it within us. Potential energy is stored energy, which stays there until something triggers or switches it on. This Eastern concept names it as 'the coiled serpent', 'serpent power' or 'Shakti' – but that doesn't say much about what it is in earthly terms.  It sounds like a spiritual concept that many probably can't relate to in our day to day reality. It has taken me years to distinguish what it is and the difference between that and other energy. I hope I can give you a starting point of understanding in what is a huge concept, in these few pages.

The experience of Kundalini that has risen is like an 'upgrade' where we feel more switched on, more conscious and aware. It can feel like a whoosh for some as it releases or a vibrating sensation, or a gentle flow by others. I experience a very mild juddering vibrating sensation through me when I wake in the morning and meditate or self-treat. For some it has been described as like a freight train running up the spine, which runs its course through the chakras, erupting like a fountain out of the crown chakra at the top of the head. The Kundalini energy is said to be (and in my experience is) stored at the base of the spine, the perineum.

When it is first triggered, activated or opened up it is sometimes likened to a red hot poker shooting up the spine. I used to feel a dull stabbing pain in my perineum when I was about 8 or 9 years, but I didn't know what it was. I would have probably just complained that I kept having a pain, as we do, until we have a framework to make sense of those experiences.  When I had homeopathy there was a tremendous force unleashed which welled up inside me to push previously stuck grief through. I howled literally and uncontrollably for 20 minutes which gave way to an incredible sense of peace that I'd felt when I'd experienced near death. The next day I could barely speak, it was slightly slurred and slow, I felt blissed out. But again, I didn't know what it was as I had no context for it. I felt that the homeopathy had shifted something within me that was stuck and needed to come out. My first reiki treatment also unleashed more as it worked on a blockage in my throat, which felt like a tangible golf ball sized lump moving up my throat. This was connected with my inability to communicate assertively.

Whether we come to realise (and release and unleash) that potential and how much actual potential we have, is our own soul journey and perhaps what we are here to experience. This energy can help people to transcend from ordinary to extraordinary when it is fully flowing through us, it can increase intelligence on mental levels as well as emotional and spiritual intelligence. It is like our supercharge or super power. It is the difference between that fast supercharge of your phone, compared to the trickle charge which takes longer. It can give us tremendous stamina. When the energy flows freely through someone they may appear to be glowing, vibrant, they may have presence, emanating radiance and peace, be exceptionally intelligent and 'switched on', the lights are on and the person is home, they are more present. Their heart shines out of their eyes. People may feel touched in their presence and not understand or know why. It is also said that you wouldn't know an enlightened man if you passed him in the street and that is a great distinction.

As the energy tries to rise up it hits blocks, and sometimes needs a bit more oomph such as that from reiki or other energy therapies to help push it through. See the section on the chakras in the energy hygiene section because these blocks – our humanness – can then cause this energy to fall back down again if we have insufficient oomph. And that's how we can stay stuck.

However, until it has run its course of cleansing and purification, we may experience a bizarre range of physical, mental and emotional symptoms. Often GPs or medical providers can find no medical cause for these and are stumped. They may diagnose spiritual and Kundalini awakenings as psychosis or mental health conditions. An interesting read on this subject is Lee Sanella's 'Psychosis or Transcendence' which I came across online shortly after I first heard about Kundalini energy and was useful for me. I was sitting in a crystal class as our tutor told us about her experience and the symptoms, as my friend looked at me and said, 'that sounds like you'. It did. I began my research and found El Collie's work online who published articles discussing the numerous symptoms she experienced.

The symptoms of fibromyalgia, such as pain and pressure sensitivity, noise sensitivity, chemical sensitivity, chronic fatigue, shooting pains and nerve pains, 'spiritual flu' (feeling like coming down with the flu then it goes), sleeping difficulty, fibro-fog (problems with memory and concentration) IBS, stiffness, depression, anxiety, headaches and so on can be very difficult to live with. However, if they are also accompanied by feelings of expansiveness, a sense of a deeper reality, crashing sounds (like a sonic boom) and white light flashing (like an old style flash bulb going off) during meditation or falling asleep, a blue light flashing in the field of vision (which isn't an optical problem), feelings of bliss and ecstasy, increased sex drive, feeling fully functioning, a great sense of wellness, increased creativity (it is our creative force) feeling whole, connected and at One with everyone and everything, colours appearing brighter and intuitive inspirations and experiences flow, it may well be an awakening.

I took hope that this was what was unfolding, not a 'dead end' of illness. In Steve Taylor's book 'From Out of the Darkness' he gives examples of how people have undergone the turmoil of spiritual awakening through various triggers resulting in their transformation. I certainly related having had a near death experience and repeated episodes of the dark night of the soul, but wasn't out of the woods yet. Russell Razzaque's book 'Breaking down is waking up', also gives hope that this is a process. It is said, and I agree, that the current pandemic will be triggering many awakenings as many believe that humanity is on the verge of the largest awakening in the history of the earth. I believe that could well be the case too. People's perception and reality is challenged by the extraordinary circumstances and confusion.

I have observed when working with people as they are awakening that one of the first stages that they experience is the emergence of fear. This can be triggered by situations such as trauma, psychic development, yoga, intense meditation and now perhaps pandemics. The fear which may already be within anyway from past experiences which have not been faced and dealt with, can be triggered in the present by current situations. This is often then projected out on to the outer situation so that hopefully the person can begin to 'see' and make sense of their inner reality and consciousness. When the person takes ownership and acceptance of their role in their life experience (it is all about me) and work through it, and let go of it, they then get to go onto the next level…ie that chakra clears, opens and the energy moves on to a clearing of the next chakra and so it goes on.

So, I found that there were many more people out there like this who had these symptoms and came through it. I found it such a hopeful perspective, rather than being something I was 'stuck with' there was something that I could work through. I wondered what my life might have been like had the GP years ago enquired about whether I was experiencing an outpouring of creativity, poetry, expansiveness and intuitive experiences. However, if that had been in my plan it would have happened and this way was the way for my soul growth, which I accept.

If you recognise any of the above symptoms, and are struggling, try to find a health practitioner or counsellor who has experience and understanding of spiritual awakenings. This may be a holistic therapist, mindfulness practitioner, energy therapist, transpersonal, gestalt or humanistic therapist. Particularly from a self-care perspective this gives us some meaning that we can come of the darkness and into the light.

## Spiritual crisis & the dark night of the soul

Opening up can throw us into disarray and chaos as the lid comes off and 'stuff' pours out, in order that we transform. It is a tough process, just like shaking one of those snow globes.

There can be layers of this over time, our development is often likened to peeling the layers of an onion. Having just emerged from another layer recently, it struck me how I knew this place now. That in itself was reassuring, instead of reactive. I had an inner map of the territory. It is the cycle of death and rebirth - not literal but for me I recognise those deep dark feelings and depressions - which some call the Dark night of the Soul. This is for me where I now know that a layer of my ego is dying, my soul is pushing through as it were, emerging arising and nudging the ego out of the way. It goes from a place of 'I know best, I'm on it' where the ego tries to control life to 'there is another way', which is the gentle way of the spirit.

The ego can shatter and crack or just dissolve as that other way, the spirit emerges, peaking its head through the ego like a daffodil trying to bloom as it emerges from the depths of the soil. It can become an internal battle if we don't understand what is going on and allow ourselves to surrender and 'go with the flow'. We may cling on desperately to the old ways because this is all we have known and change is frightening. This is a process of trust (in the process of life or a higher power, or God) when we can surrender to the process, and the ego yields and lets go. As we may come to know or revisit this place over time and get to know that route, there is assurance that there is something better the other side of our darkness, that out of the void comes the light.

## The suicide response

It is often at this point that I believe people become suicidal, because they feel instinctively that there is a 'death', a dying of something. In the confusion and pain of that place, instead of trusting that it is the ego dying and a process which, given time (law of impermanence), can be worked through, they misguidedly feel that they have to act on those thoughts and feelings of suicide. Having been in that place time and time again now over the years, I can see it, but not so in the early years whilst in it. It is undoubtedly very dark, raw and painful. However, the darker the night, the brighter the starlight.

Understanding what is going on is key and I not so long back realised that years ago I would have been hospitalised. This time, with different tools, self-care was prominent. I took an extra day a week off, I took myself on long walks, I practised kindfulness and self-compassion, as much as I know how. I went away to give myself breaks (and gave thanks with gratitude that instead of being hospitalised, I could feel 'the balm of nature as my salve'). I accepted the process and felt gratitude at how much I have learnt over the years. So we can get there!

## The gift of the present

Meditation over the years in its various forms, has allowed and taught me to better practise present moment awareness as I go about my daily life - apart from where my keys are! I find that quite ironic and symbolic that I misplace 'the keys'. By the time my focus and awareness stays on them more frequently and I mindfully know where I have put them, I may well have the key to my consciousness! However for now they remind me of the key to compassion and not to judge my inability to be present more often!

I think it is important to remember this, as Jon Kabatt Zin says *'Meditation is not relaxation spelled differently. This doesn't mean that meditation is not frequently accompanied by profound relaxation and by deep feelings of well-being. Of course, it can be sometimes. But mindfulness meditation is the embrace of any and all mind states in awareness, without preferring one to another. From the point of view of mindfulness practise, pain or anguish or for the matter boredom or impatience or frustration or anxiety or tension or tension in the body are all equally valid objects of our attention if we find them arising in the present moment, each a rich opportunity for insight and learning and potentially, for liberation, rather than signs that our meditation practice is not succeeding, because we are feeling relaxed or experiencing calmness or bliss in some moment.'*

# The key!

Accepting what is happening in the here and now. Meditation isn't about emptying your mind as I've said, it is about just allowing what comes up to surface or emerges, breathing into it and allowing it to be without judging it. My right buttock is hurting sitting here, but it is as it is. It is a sensation, it will pass, it won't be there forever. Pain does come and go and when I detach from it, rather than ruminating and clinging on to my 'ouch that hurts', we can say, 'there's the pain', witnessing that it is there, rather than becoming it and it can subside.

Detaching - or de-aching as I see it - from our thoughts and feelings is about not attaching meaning to them. I had an epiphany this week when working with a client who doesn't communicate verbally and has reactive, reflexive behaviours. Usually I take my glasses off before the treatment as the client can grab things around them. I forgot this time and suddenly found them being swiped! The client's nails caught my skin and it hurt. I allowed myself to feel that sensation of pain and tuned in to acknowledge my own feelings about it, whilst calmly saying 'no' to the client. I felt shocked, it had happened quite quickly; I breathed to let it go.

It was a profound realisation that I could let it go so easily because their behaviour was a reflex reaction rather than personal, it wasn't about me, they didn't intend to hurt me. In that, it brought a tear of gratitude to my eyes because I could see how often I did attach meaning to other people's behaviours, which then caused me to cling on to them to some degree or another. When we can detach and see that it often isn't personal we can let go. Similar in meditation, when we learn not to judge the mind straying or the thoughts or feelings that we have, they are as they are, it's the nature of the mind, we build a more compassionate practise both in meditation and in our present moment.

## A realistic session

And breath... chitter chatter mind, oh this chair is hard, my bum aches, I'm a bit hungry, oh an itch..I may have beans for my tea, I fancy those, where am I going on holiday this year... and back we go to the breath... I'm going to see Gloria later, we may go for a... Oh my breath, breathe... I quite fancy a cake... oh Breath DraT! I'm rubbish at this, why can't I do it... you are already doing it... back to the breath... I'm feeling frustration, rage... grrr... that's OK, notice it, breath, it'll pass, back to the breath...

So we will have many, many times where we are side-tracked, where our focus goes astray, and from this I feel that I learn. It isn't because we're doing it wrong, I don't think you can do it wrong, but many of us feel that way about meditation. We complicate it, by our nature. Sit, focus on the breath, mind stray, back to the breath... mind stray for many many moments, oh my mind's gone again, it's OK, back to the breath... oh gosh, my mind went for a complete holiday from the breath then, it's OK, back to the breath... ding... the bell to signify the end... oh crumbs, my mind has been straying so much... It's OK, it is as it is, some days are like this... keep showing up for the next day and the next day.

## The business of busyness

STOP! Create some space for you. Block out part of your diary. Give yourself the gift of some time. Easier said than done, I totally appreciate.

When I went through a period of being very busy at work, I'd find that instead of sticking to my opening hours, I would book people in later on in the day, past my closing time. I was increasingly doing this and on one occasion when I came home at 4.30pm, it was a relief to come home at a decent time. I blocked off 'ME time' in my diary after work with a big ME label to remind myself that I mattered too. Putting it into practise was challenging sometimes, especially if I went into fear that I needed to keep doing to earn my living or I was concerned about someone else's wellbeing if I couldn't fit them in. I did book some appointments in still, but with more awareness of checking in to see how I felt and asking myself 'did I have the energy?' rather than just doing it automatically.

I also found that I was in the habit of forcing my diary and time. If there were gaps in it, what would I do with the time. I'd put efforts in to advertise or send out special offers to fill the slots and also verge on panic about it, rather than thinking it's time to do admin (as much as I tried to tell myself that initially). The thought of me 'waiting around' for half an hour or an hour for another client was unthinkable.

# Gaps that need to be filled

This went back to when as a child 'doing nothing' was boring. Constant stimulation was a distraction for the pain underneath that threatened to well up if it was lacking, so wasn't an option - time had to be filled rather than felt. It was a gap that needed to be filled and that's OK until we are ready to go there and allow that gap to be as it is and fill ourselves with it.

First, up must come those painful emotions to be dealt with. So often we will keep on keeping on until we are in the right place to do that. If you recognise that this is probably true for you, it may be advisable to have some therapy to give yourself the space to allow those feelings to emerge.

The irony is, the universe hates a void. So when we give something up and create a void, our ego mind may rush to fill that gap, as mine had. That mechanism can be there to 'put a lid' on something, to keep it down. The ego seeks to protect us, but isn't always right, much as it likes to think that it is. However, if we can surrender and trust the Powers that Be (Let go and let God), that void is very often filled with something nicer. I tend to find that when I give something up, whether it's planning as in this case or sugar in another, there may be an initial wobble whereby I may feel teary or emotional or panicky as something like 'old negativity' is released, but as I progress, something better such as more peace or calmer feelings come in. Now I accept that God plans my diary, I trust that those that need treatments will come, I will be supported financially by the abundance of the Universe and that I have been given the gift of time at these points in order to do something else. I tune in to find out what that is, is it to cleanse and clear my therapy room, to do some admin to send some texts or reply to calls. Or just to be and go home and have a nice cup of tea, before the next round.

## Doing mode

I also realised around that time that I was finding concentration very difficult again, whereas previously through meditation it had improved significantly. Before meditation (and Reiki) my thoughts went at 50,000 miles per hour, and after, they now go at just 20,000 mph. If we are in doing mode, our brains can end up getting overloaded and overwhelmed with information. 'Being' helps us to process information. Those gaps in my diary were there for a reason, that I came to learn.   Lock down !

But for now, I couldn't focus on reading and I couldn't sit and just watch TV, I'd be up and down doing other things. My mind was going ten to the dozen and before I realised it I was thinking about other things and had missed the plot and had no idea what was going on, whilst thinking about things that I had to do. This wasn't a great loss in many ways as I'm not overly keen on much of what's on TV, but it can have it's uses for relaxing, unwinding and switching off. Many people sit and do something whilst watching the TV to engage that 'doing' part of them, like knitting, that keeps them busy. My aim was to follow my work motto, 'just be'.

My meditative practise at that time was also more 'on the go'. With doing Reiki self healing, I was still doing something and with mindful running or walking, it was 'doing' I didn't want to sit still and 'be'. Sometimes, as mentioned previously, it can be that we are avoiding something and we may choose to work through that.

Sitting and listening to ourselves may allow something to surface and emerge, a memory or thought or a feeling of what we are trying to escape from, through busyness. Or some may say it is part of their way of being and 'if it ain't broke don't fix it' which is right for them. The way that I dealt with it then was, 'it is as it is, for now'. If you are a doer, what's it about for you? Are you OK with it? Do you feel like you have a choice in what you are doing? Do you feel resentful because you don't feel like you have so much to do and you are the only one that can do it?

I knew I'd get that nudge to sit and look within if it were the case as I do believe in 'right timing' that we instinctively know when the time is right to make changes. 'Doing', for me, was obviously serving a function on some level at that point that I would probably learn something from. Sometimes it can have a habit of highlighting the opposite. I've been cultivating a more disciplined practise recently, to look at and work through my own resistances, it feels right and the Right Time in my heart to do that now. So trust!

## I don't have the time

Probably one of the most difficult challenges to overcome and one which also goes hand in hand with resistance, discipline and priorities. I guess it can also come down at root level to: do you want to make the time for it? We may think that we do, because we'd benefit or 'need' it or it'll help us and that may be so. Or it might be that there is a block there of not really wanting that subconsciously. There are the obvious solutions such as 'set your alarm, get up ten minutes earlier', but how do you respond to that? Is the resistance still there? An approach might be to sit in contemplation and try the looking within method and ask for inspiration, what your blocks are, and a way forward that is right for you.

## Types of meditation

There are so many forms of meditation. A good place to start is to download a free app such as Insight Timer or another popular one is Headspace. Have a look on Youtube for various guided meditations. You could also try looking at pictures of mandalas with beautiful music and also listening to special music which deepens meditation and takes us into deeper states of relaxation, sometimes known as binaural beats in that it is said to affect the brain waves when listening to it via headphones. I've found it effective.

Transcendental meditation is a practise wherein that person may be trying to empty their mind, as they are trying to access 'the gap' in between thoughts. This can allow the person to connect with higher states of consciousness, or the reservoir of energy and creativity.

Mantras are another form of meditation, such as 'Ohm', or 'So hum' maybe used and chanting and singing phrases link us with deeper states, such as the particular favourite of mine 'Om namah shiva'. These are also ways of approaching meditation and can be very joyful, especially in groups.

I liken the practise of Reiki, particularly self-healing, to being a meditative process. When we are giving Reiki, we step aside from the 'outcome', we let the energy flow through us, we don't attach to a result (never promise that it can cure or heal, as this can be false hope), but just notice the sensations and the flow, not judging or interpreting what this means, I just allow it to flow through me as if I am a drainpipe. With the self-treating, there is no 'other', so this is more focused again. This can be done whilst lying down in 'corpse' pose, during a series of meditations called Hatsu Rei Ho, or intuitively. As we practise Reiki, or receive it, our brainwaves are thought to be akin to the theta state, which is a state of relaxation similar to being on the edge of sleep or wakefulness.

The benefits of a focused meditation is primarily cultivating more discipline and retraining the mind. This was and still is my journey. By focusing on the breath as we breath in and out, chanting mantras or observing a candle flicker and looking at or becoming the flame, then noticing that whenever our thoughts stray to other things, we become more attentive and aware of our 'monkey mind'. Noticing when the thoughts stray from the present moment, and catching ourselves and bringing ourselves back to the task in hand, can help us to exercise and train the 'mind muscle'. Through this we may develop the ability to deepen our focus and concentration in our general lives more as well as be aware of the beauty of the present moment, which really is a gift.

# Chapter Fourteen

## The answers are within

### Defining intuition

The definition of intuition from the Oxford English Dictionary is: "*The ability to understand or know something immediately, without conscious reasoning.*"

Those who are intuitive often have a high degree of sensitivity and awareness. It may seem like they have a sixth sense. I think of it as my 'inner tuition' or my 'inner guide' and it has been at the forefront of teaching me how to self-care better. Through that, it has helped my healing journey tremendously; it is my internal navigation system.

Long before I even realised what it was, it was guiding me, as yours too may be guiding you. When I was sixteen I received a very clear message from my intuition advising me 'never take any drugs other than cannabis and certainly not LSD'. It was a gut feeling and huge knowing. I just accepted it, even though I didn't really know what it was. It just happened to me from time to time; I thought it happened to everyone; I believe it does, to varying degrees, and I'm not alone in thinking that our sixth sense is our lost sense. I often wonder (and know) how different the world would be, if we learnt to listen to and trust it more. No more bullshit! It would force people to become more honest and take better responsibility if they knew that others could see straight through them.

## 14. The Answers Are Within

Learning to listen (and argue with!) my intuition has been a journey for me which, along with meditation, has helped me to connect back to my true self. I think of intuition as communication from my soul, the spiritual part of me, my spirit, or my 'higher self'. It is my 'inner tuition', there to guide me, to help me along my path and when I listen to it, it can help to smooth things and make some things a little easier along the way which is a great tool for self-care. Bluntly put, it can cut through the crap!

I believe that we all have intuition, but because we aren't taught to use it or listen to it, it can get buried and we may not be aware of it. Think of all the cars that are on the road and a new make comes out. You know nothing about cars, you're not particularly bothered and don't really care, so don't pay any attention at all, but there it is driving around. A friend then points out this new car - suddenly you see them everywhere. They are there, just as your intuition is, it's just that you aren't aware of it and haven't paid it much attention. There it is, hiding from us in plain sight!

This was true for me. When Sue felt that my issues were a result of psychic imbalances, because she'd developed her abilities, she could see it clearly in me (as I see and feel it in others) but I couldn't at that point see it within myself. I looked back at the times when I was younger that I'd had a strong inner knowing that something was going to happen, such as a boyfriend at the time going off with a friend, which was complete unexpected! Another boyfriend going to end the relationship. Seeing how boys in my class at school would change and look as they got older. Why had I been strongly drawn to learn from a library book how to do palm readings at the school fair, for something different to offer to do to fundraise, yet people had said it was good? How had I known these things and many more? I didn't think I was 'psychic' as she'd said I was, that was surely something people did on phone lines?! But I did think that there was something going on that was worthy of my attention and since owning and acknowledging it, and putting it to the test to prove it to myself, I came to see that there was something in this - which did blow my mind literally! And semantically, I have always preferred the word intuitive as I feel that while the word psychic does set us apart, we can all be, by our very nature, intuitive.

Intuition is said to work from the right side of the brain, the creative side, which operates the left side of the body and equates with the feminine aspect, our receptive, 'being', feeling side. The right side of the body is said to relate to the left brain, our logical, masculine aspect and 'doing'. Our intuition develops through a mode of 'being' and acceptance of what is. We access intuition through stillness and relaxation. However, to be 'whole' brained, and therefore balanced and grounded, I believe that we benefit from acting on our intuition through our 'doing', masculine mode. This helps us to integrate the knowing and 'walk our talk', keeping both feet on the ground. Meditation is the first base for intuitive development and the looking within exercise later in the chapter can help you with that too. We benefit from quietening the mind in order to hear our inner voice or notice our inner-sight (insight) more clearly.

## The conscious, subconscious and super conscious

The superconscious or collective unconscious as the psychologist Jung describes it, where our intuition can reside, is sometimes known as the collective conscious or to others known as the Akashic records. It is said to be that which links to all; it is the 'greater mind' to which we are all connected via our Higher Self or soul. Being connected to our Higher Self helps us to cut through confusion a lot quicker: this is where our answers lie and where our own pure, uninfluenced, personal truth about our lives (our life map) is said to exist. Our Higher Self acts like a messenger as it is always connected to the answers which reside in the collective unconscious or Akashic records, but it isn't always easy to hear or feel the connection to our Higher Self or our intuition if we have issues in the way.

## Recognising your intuition: ways in which our intuition can make itself known

Think of the first fleeting thought e.g. on immediate sight of someone, before they have even introduced themselves or told you what they want you to hear. This is how people project their persona, 'their mask' out onto the world, which may not be the full truth. We can all do it for various reasons, often on some level to just keep ourselves safe until we learn a more authentic way of being. Your intuition may blurt something out such as 'I don't like them', or you may feel your gut drop. We can consciously check in with our intuition on first meeting someone and listen for what it says. It could be 'that person reminds me of such and such a person' (which may be transference, or maybe similarity), or 'I don't like this person' or 'I feel totally at ease, very open, safe, and completely able to be myself with this person' or 'steer clear of this person', etc.

Sometimes we may doubt our first thoughts and impressions but if we give it time, it might be that we were right (or wrong!) Wait and see. Some say you can't go by first impressions; I disagree in my experience and listening to it could even be life-saving – but that is my experience, check in with yours.

It is worth noting that discernment 'notices'; it's an observation and we can remain open to the possibility that something is so, not assuming ourselves to be right (the need to be right comes from the ego). Judgement of another is something that is condemning and we often do so through our own fear. We close our energy up and remain fixed, static, rigid and stuck to our answer – this judgement is thus not (solely) intuition, but ego. When we discern what our first impressions of intuition are, we can then listen to our inner-tuition on 'how to proceed' as the interaction unfolds – or not. It's pretty much like noticing how someone is 'in our opinion', deciding whether to interact or not, then either walking away or deciding whether to dip our toe in the water and see how it unfolds.

Intuition can come as a knowing – we don't know how we know, but we do know with a great assurance that e.g. the relationship your best friend is embarking upon will not work out, or 'they don't look good together' (look like a mismatch). We may just know that the job is right for us. That knowing may come from the whole of our being, or our heart or a gut feeling.

Inspirational a-ha! moments – sudden knowing, realisations and understandings. Perhaps also felt as 'inner leaps, jumps or pings' as the light-bulb goes on. They tend to feel energetically 'high', excitable such as energy rises, full of energy and enlivened. Penny drop moments, such as 'this is the way to proceed with the situation'.

We may feel very drawn to a person, like a magnetic pull. Interest or captivation (not obsession) accompanied by positive feelings. This can also be to a pull to a place, feeling drawn to a particular town or a house. Can be characterised by a feeling of 'fascination', wonder and awe which comes in repeatedly as nudges or prompts.

Gut dropping moments can be where the energy just drops and we feel tired or drained. We may feel repelled, like we want to get away. Alarm bells and red flags can be experienced as a startled feeling, a shocked feeling, a 'head's up' to 'Pay Attention!'. Have you ever ignored the alarm bells and made excuses for a person or justified their actions? The classic abuse situation. We knew something wasn't right all along. Why didn't we listen to our intuition?

Sometimes it is an internal feeling which some people call a 'head's up' to pay attention and listen to what someone else is saying. I have this as an inner nudge, an awareness that what this person is saying is important, relevant to me and makes sense and could be useful to me or another I may come across.Their intuitive energy is purer and higher (doesn't come from ego which is lower) which is knocking on the door of my spirit, what they are saying raises me up. 'Oh?!'

Noticing that many different, unrelated people are saying the same thing to you within a short space of time e.g. 'you will get better' if you have been ill. I really appreciate these intuitive genuine messages from people, because often people are unaware that they are giving them and they are given in all innocence rather than from a place of power or ego. I was going through a period of self-doubt not so long back, which I either take to supervision or talk to a close friend about - I never mention this to clients per se and attend to my energy. However, I spontaneously received a few lovely reviews and a few clients mentioned how grateful they were for the treatments that they'd received. It really did seem like the universe was saying, 'come on Emma, it's just a blip, it's all fine!'

It maybe a 'hunch' or a discomfort that 'something's not quite right' e.g. before we take a trip somewhere, plans seem to go awry or are difficult to make (or I'm trying to buy something online and the transaction won't go through). We might not know why or how. At the start of January I tried to get quoted for the kitchen to be done, but it was really difficult for me get this done. Looking back, the timing would not have been right as we later went into lockdown. As we did come out of lockdown, everything flowed smoothly. Intuition may also transpire as a gut instinct that 'something is going to happen'. Ominous feelings or feelings of doom (once own negativity has been addressed) may accompany this.

Our intuition can present as an image – a picture flashing up in our mind's eye (3rd eye) or overlaying something or someone, so they may appear to be different to how you know they usually are. Their appearance may change in some way. Often we may have an image and say 'I can see that.' (or 'I can't see that'), or 'I have a lovely image of you…'.

Sometimes I will have a repetitive thought – a recurring thought, or a niggling feeling which keeps coming back. It can be a name of a person, a name of a place, a route to work or even a song. This often occurs 'at the back of the mind'. If its a song I will sometimes google the words and see if there's a message in there for me.

Many of us are sensitive to atmospheres. This can be a strange or odd feeling or sensation when we walk into a room, an area (such as a town new to us), or a place or we meet a new person. 'This place gives me the creeps'; 'that person makes me feel sick' (or we may shudder around them).

'Take note' is something for me that is similar to dictation. I will hear a line of words running through my head, often lovely, wise words, which demand to be written down. Sometimes it's been an image which impulsively I might want to create. This is sometimes known as channelling and may link to our soul or other beings in other realms or dimensions, such as spirit helpers, or ascended beings, or angels according to our beliefs. I find that they are first and foremost teachings for me, but to also be shared with others.

Our inner voice may give clear intuitive guidance. It firmly says, 'drive that way today' or 'lock the door' or 'get another set of car keys cut' or 'slow down' or 'don't date that person'. This was very clear instruction for me (as was my argument for cake instead from my ego!) that you can read about in the Animal chapter, and my experience with the horse Thom.

When doing therapy work, therapists will often have an intuitive feeling which transpires as being drawn to or having a pull towards a certain part of the body, e.g. the knee, which directs us where to work.

An awareness of when someone is lying – hearing something within someone's voice or a slight discomfort that for some reason what the person is saying is not ringing true; there is lack of authenticity and the person does not seem genuine – we just don't 'get it' and it doesn't feel right. This is also similar to when there is an awareness of what someone's motives or intentions are, other than what they portray e.g. they may say that they are 'only joking' but there is a nasty undertone or vibe going on.

Brightening is where something looks brighter, more obvious and it can 'leap out' on a visual level, eg a book on a shelf, often accompanied by feeling drawn to it and a kind of excitement and a glow of light. The item seems energised, almost as if it's waving to us, 'choose me!' This is how I chose the first spiritual books that I bought and which are still my favourite 'Spiritual Intelligence' and 'White Eagle'; there are beautiful words in both which truly nourished me.

I also have sudden urges or impulses which make no sense to me on a logical level, such as 'I must watch that programme on quantum physics, even though I have no idea what it's about! However, when I watch it I receive inspiration and teaching and suddenly something about it makes sense in relation to what I do. I also get sent to the cinema this way, just recently to teach me more about shadow aspects of characters in films and how this occurs in 'real life' too.

## Increasing our consciousness and awareness

What is Your Favourite Colour and why? What does that colour mean to you?

If someone asks this and we reply 'I don't know' it is because we are unconscious or unaware of the reason; it is our 'blind spot' and we can't see why. One of the goals of intuitive development is to develop and attain consciousness, in order for us to evolve as a human and spiritual being – to be aware of ourselves e.g. 'I feel drawn to blue because it helps me to feel peaceful and calm'. We can access information like this by listening to our 'still, small voice', by looking within and practising meditation. Everyone's consciousness can be restricted and closed through fear. This takes us back to meditation to quiet the mind and find our answers through our inner support system.

Development is sometimes called 'opening up'. Our mind opens up; our consciousness and awareness expands. This is why someone who is primarily logical and left brained, may be seen to closed or narrow minded and not as intuitive. They may be less feeling orientated, having suppressed those or be fixed - however they also have many other valuable skills such as being grounded, academic, commonsensical, focused and logical. Balanced awareness would endeavour to cultivate all of these traits for the whole brained approach. A year or so after I started meditating, I had a very interesting experience where I felt a rush of energy (as movement) in my brain, in the centre. Whether it is the case or not, I don't know, but to me it felt like my 'whole brain' was opening up, that a doorway between the left and right, or a wall, was coming down. When I am practising meditation in a more focused way, I also find that I get white light flashing inside my brain, often just before I drop off to sleep (like an old style flashbulb going off) and a noise like an old style flashbulb boom.

## Obstacles and barriers to intuition

Our intuition flows better in the moment, when we don't question it and just let it come, so if you feel that you are onto something, if you feel that connection, just let it come, let it flow. Questioning uses the logical rational mind and halts the flow of intuition. This is not to say that we shouldn't question, I always have one foot in sceptic, but it is about knowing when to and when not to question. Let the intuition come/flow – then question afterwards. Be sceptical; be rational as well as using your intuition, I believe this attitude of curiosity leads to a wholistic, whole-person, whole-brained approach.

## 14. The Answers Are Within

Sometimes a fear of being right is downright scary! What would happen if we were right? We may fear the change which listening to our intuition would bring. Sometimes we may fear being wrong; we may fear failing. We may have to do things differently; that can be scary. Addressing our fears where we can helps us to let go of them, which opens us up further.

People pleasing can be an obstacle in expressing our intuition e.g. if we feel that by trusting our intuition and acting on it, we risk disappointing or feeling that we will hurt someone else. We then block our intuition. Cultural or religious beliefs may also cause us to keep our intuition dampened down, believing it to come from evil spirits or the devil, or that others will accuse us of this, reminiscent of the witch hunts in the past. There was a very real reason to keep things suppressed, for fear of our lives.

Emotional stress makes it very difficult to hear our intuition when we are feeling confused. The noise of our emotions and the chatter of our minds can cause us to be out of tune, like interference of our reception – or a radio between two stations. Emotions cause the same noise!

Right timing is important to acknowledge, as sometimes we don't have the answers in that moment because certain things have yet to come to light. We may not have all the information just yet. We don't always arrive at the crossroads when the lights are on green, sometimes we have to wait a while on red – and be patient. When in doubt, don't.

Our physical & material needs can cause a block for us. Paying attention to 'earthly matters' mean that it can be harder to hear the voice of our intuition and also during illness or a crisis (though crisis may trigger and open it up for others). These times can also be times of learning. Over the years and with time and practise, the more in tune you become the less out of tune you get during these periods of earthly learning.

Attaching to an outcome can be a solid wall sometimes, when we want something too much, the voice of our ego, or our lower self, can drown out our intuition. 'I want this, I want that' and our energy is invested (paying attention is an energy investment) on the end result and what we want to attain. When we focus on the present, we are paying attention to the here and now and we are more likely to notice our intuition.

Do you recognise any of these instances where your intuition was trying to speak to you but you didn't listen or couldn't hear?

## When we get things wrong

This can be very similar to our blocks. Try looking within and asking yourself why you got that wrong? Listen for your answer.

With relief I took much pressure off myself by realising that we don't always get it right - no one does! By viewing 'mistakes' as opportunities for learning and growth we can learn from them. By taking responsibility for our own errors we allow ourselves to grow as a person. We then may also be less hard on ourselves, when we think we've got it wrong and instead cultivate a degree of acceptance for 'going with the flow' and accepting what just is.

## 14. The Answers Are Within

When we have asked a question and heard yes or no, it can help to check in with our heart to see whether it feels open or closed (is there a feeling of being expansive and open or tight shut in the heart area?) as this can give us a measure of whether we are able to remain open to something, without feeling fear. Does our heart feel comfortable about this answer? Our expectations can often override our intuition. If we can let go of the outcome and trust that we always 'get what we need', or trust in the Divine Plan or in fate, we may be able to hear the intuition still. When we get scared of making the wrong decision and go into fear, it can again cause us to overly focus on the outcome instead of staying in the moment.

Sometimes we can 'push the river'. Our desires keep us swimming up stream; we may be too eager because we wanted something and actually push it away. Perhaps our timing wasn't right, and we were impatient and tried to make things happen before they were naturally 'ripe' and ready to occur and fall into place. We may be trying to control 'the flow' instead of going with it.

If we are depressed or in a negative frame of mind, it can cloud our mind and cloud our judgement making it very difficult to see or hear our intuition. When we have irrational fear within such as insecurity we can tense and close up to protect ourselves, making it difficult to remain open and see with clarity. This comes back to purification of our mental processes. This is noticing and working through the way that we think and what we think of ourselves and others, looking at our issues and our emotional baggage, and paying attention to physical needs. These are all areas which serve us to address along the path of intuitive development.

## Is it my imagination?

The imagination is said to be one step away from intuition and a question that is frequently asked 'how do I know that it's not my imagination?' We don't always know and the thing with developing our intuition is, because everyone is different, we have to work out what works best for us. It's like a puzzle; you may be given the pieces of the jigsaw but you have to put it together yourself to find out how it works for you – often 'getting it wrong' along the way, which can show us more about what it means to get it 'right'.

Usually, if it is not our imagination, the 'intuition' will keep coming back, the thought or feeling will come again e.g. that 'niggling feeling'. I once said during a course that my Mum came on, 'just make it up as you go along', i.e. feel into the intuition and take it step by step. If it is your imagination, go with the flow and see what transpires. She took it to mean lie! I explained it further, it is about being honest and saying to another if it involves another, 'I'm not sure if this is my imagination, but I'm going to explore it on the basis that it might be my intuition'. Mindfully lying and being manipulative can often be counter productive with intuition, because it works like an 'off' switch to the higher intuitive processes.

## The benefits of developing your intuition

The personal benefits of developing our intuition are many. It can help our life run a little more smoothly, increase our inner confidence, enhance and speed up the decision-making process. It can help to build self-trust and thereby helps us to trust others too, It can help to cut through confusing circumstances quicker than we previously have. It helps us to stay in the now; to focus on the present. The process teaches us to honour and respect ourselves and in that we can find a more solid sense of self-esteem, and self-worth. It brings honour to others too as we learn to respect that because we have our own individual differences, so too do others. It can help to increase our understanding of others, and ourselves, which promotes more harmonious relationships and inner peace. Our concentration may improve and with that the memory too.

# Being realistic

Developing your intuition does not mean that we will have all the answers; sometimes life is very confusing and painful. This is a journey and intuitive development rarely happens overnight. It can be a long, slow, arduous, frustrating process at times, though at other times you may come on in leaps and bounds. Life still goes on with its ups and downs and its moments of clarity and blind spots. No one is right 100% of the time. This would be too easy. What would we learn?

If you find that you are becoming unbalanced and ungrounded it may help you to temporarily stop all intuitive/ spiritual practises. Focus on more logical practises e.g. a game of sudoku, or get grounded and go for a walk in nature.

The integration of intuitive or spiritual information with logic often leads to what is sometimes referred to as the 7th sense, the all important Common Sense! To progress intuitively is about developing emotionally, mentally and spiritually as well, It is about aiming to be balanced on all four levels.

# Strengthening your intuition

Meditation, as I've said, helps to quieten the mind and the mental chatter in order to be able to hear the still, small voice. If the mind is chattering, perhaps it is trying to tell us something – if we can't sleep at night because thoughts are going round in our heads, are we paying enough attention to them during the day or is the noise of the TV or radio a distraction from our own thoughts? Sitting in meditation or mindfully contemplating an issue and giving ourselves a fixed period of time to think can clear the mind. Other forms of meditation can help to discipline the mind to focus more keenly, for example focusing and looking at a candle.

*Pay attention to your intuition.* Listen to it; notice your inner voice speaking to you. This might sound very obvious, but how often do we not pay attention to our intuition? Attention is energy, we give it energy, so when we pay attention to our intuition we are plugging it in and charging it, powering it up! Similarly, by acting on our intuition we are paying attention to it which grounds it in reality. This naturally strengthens it and with this action we may find that we can cut through confusing circumstances quicker than we have done in the past (with the benefit of hindsight). e.g. 'lock the door now' (stops the burglar), 'back up the computer' (computer then blows up).

*Personal development* - as we clear away our own issues and blocks we create a better flow; we clear the way for more intuitive energy and information to flow through. Doing this in groups or being in a circle, by being around other people who are intuitive or focusing on their development can have a synergistic effect on intuitive development. It helps to amplify and strengthen it as often these are positive 'inspirational' people who enjoy inspiring others too. Sitting regularly, usually weekly, in a development circle helps to develop intuitive abilities

Creativity naturally opens up our intuition, so drawing and painting may take on new dimensions. Journaling can help too, plus writing 'free-flow' – sitting down and writing EVERYTHING that comes into the mind, no matter how irrational, disjointed or odd it may be. Do not judge yourself, do not scrutinise it, nor analyse it – the paper is a way of getting things out. When finished, throw it away. Also drawing with the non-dominant hand can free up the flow. Try also drawing emotions, and doing your own art therapy which does not have to be a masterpiece (a scribble can depict anger for instance).

Working with crystals such as amethyst, sodalite blend logic with intuition and are good starter crystals. Azurite can be used for channelling. Apophyllite and citrine are good for gut intuition and can be placed on the solar plexus, or for claircognisance placed on the crown. Kyanite connects us to spirit guides and enhances telepathy. Labadorite and moonstone help with women's intuition. Crystals are beautiful and inspiring to look at, while holding one during meditation or carrying a tumble stone can be incredibly opening.

Practising Reiki regularly has not only helped me to quieten my mind but helped with focus and concentration which naturally helps us to open up. The actual attunements to Reiki or other healing systems & modalities work as initiations which are opening, as they open up the chakras, the meridians or nadis (our energy pathways) and also keep them clear so that we can receive information.

Journaling is a valuable process of making a note of what we have experienced. For some people writing helps to consolidate information, it brings it all together and helps process and makes sense of what they are learning, plus we can then look back on it to check how accurate we were if we make a note of readings and journeys.

Good advice that I was given by a friend of mine was "stop listening to people who have their own issues and begin to listen to your spirit". What a lovely, empowering thought. As I have said, people will always give us their opinion through the filter of their own experiences and perception. Only we can truly know our own.

## Intuitive guidelines

*Tuning in* - The key to beginning to tune into our intuition is to decide for ourselves what we believe intuition to be. This involves us listening to ourselves, taking time to be quiet and still within in order to hear ourselves and begin to listen to ourselves – and to trust ourselves. We are all different and that's OK.

*Come back to your Self and 'tune' in.* You are in control of yourself and can make the decisions. It is about paying close attention to your own senses and what feels right for you; it is all about noticing what is going on for you inside – do you feel comfortable? Do you feel happy with this? How does your body feel? Try getting into your body, and out of your head.

*Talk to lots of different people* – ask them about their experiences and what they think intuition is (or whatever you want their opinion on) then consciously come back to your Self and tune into your intuition to decide what feels right for you and what makes sense to you.

*Consciously listening to yourself* - It may benefit you to begin to consciously listen to yourself if you are in the habit of 'parroting'. Within the instance of parroting you are handing over your power and control to another person and not taking responsibility. What do you think or how do you feel? Take note of *you*. Make a decision whether you are 'this or that' and own it. Your intuition is all about you! It is not about what someone else thinks – it's about listening and paying attention to you which is how we come to value ourselves. It doesn't matter one iota if someone is seemingly more experienced and knows more than you think you do, if something doesn't feel right then it isn't right for you, at least at that point in time. Through listening to our intuition, we learn to listen to ourselves in the moment and we take control of our lives and ourselves by taking back our sense of personal power. Some of what others say may be meaningful; some may not. Take what you need and dismiss the rest.

*Put your new beliefs into action:* applying your intuition and intuitive thoughts and acting on them (as long as you do no harm). As I've said, this helps to ground your intuition into experience. However, if something doesn't work for you, find another way; experiment.

*There are many paths up the same mountain.* We are all different and due to differing perceptions and experiences we 'see' things differently. What is 'pink' to one person may be 'magenta' to another. Our mental processes and experiences will affect how we perceive and and how we 'receive' things. It's not to say that another is wrong if they perceive things in a different way to us, they will likely be right for the experiences that they encounter, or want to encounter for their soul growth and those differences are all part of life's rich tapestry.

*Do no harm* – your intuition would never tell you to harm yourself or anyone else. With intuitive development comes a responsibility, for your Self. No longer do we blame others, instead we begin to take responsibility for ourselves. Sometimes this is very hard; it can be very tough, sometimes painful, to notice our shadow sides and our imperfections and take responsibility for our choices in life. Clearing our issues enables us to see more clearly and function as a purer channel for receiving intuitive information.

*Be true to ourselves.* This means acting our on intuition. This encourages us to be more honest with ourselves and others too. By honest expression, this can increase the love and understanding in our life; it brings us closer to people because we aren't hiding behind an outer mask. It allows people to know us, instead of the façade we may present to impress others because we fear being our true selves. It causes us to look and listen to the thoughts and feelings that our true Self presents and in that we get to know ourselves. What better route to self-care than being intuitively guided to what is right for us. The higher self is aware of the bigger picture, trusting that plan and letting the spirit lead as the ego steps aside, can lead to much growth, strength and resilience.

# Chapter Fifteen

## Wholesome Nutrition

### (Whole-Sum) nutrition

Nutrition has always been something that made a lot of sense to me, after all what we put in to our body powers us. The analogy of the car and not putting the right petrol or oil in and expecting it to perform well illustrates what a difference that which we put in can make to us. Although it does make sense to me, I too have my challenges nutritionally, with weight and sugar addiction which in turn teaches me more, and also helps to inform my work.

Wholesome nutrition for self-care would ideally be home cooked, home prepared fresh food, organic or home grown, additive free and local food where possible. Few of us are able to live by this ideal, with demands like raising children and working. An 80/20 rule is something more achievable to aim for for those of us who are more able. That is, eating a healthy balanced diet 80% of the time and 20% of the time acknowledging there are things that we do enjoy which might not benefit us as much.

However, if even that is too much, starting small and making small changes can still make a substantial difference. Rome was not built in a day, it can be hard to change and we also need to bear in mind that change can also be very gradual and accumulate in strength over time as we cultivate new habits. We may find that we go back to an old one and notice how it isn't serving us, we then try the new ones again and notice how good it feels, then go back to old ways, and learn from that back and forth process until better habits become more habitual. It's about doing the best that we can and acknowledging that. Beating ourselves up and feeling guilty about it will not help, see Toxic Guilt. There are some 'quick fix' things that we can do to strike more of a balance if we feel that we are lacking aptitude for self-feeding care.

## Gut feelings

You may be aware of current guidelines about cutting down on sugar, lessening intake of saturated fat and eating more monounsaturated fats, getting 25-30g of dietary fibre, having five fruit or vegetables a day (450g), eating oily fish a couple of times a week to name a few of the current guidelines. There's also the traffic light system on food packaging telling us which foods are high in fats, salt or sugar, by indicating in red and a green colour for the ones which are good to go with.

It is wise to remember that we are all different and all have different needs and striking the balance is also about working out what seems to suit us personally. It is a fine dance between listening to our own bodies and experiences as well as listening to the current guidelines. It will always be a bit of a guessing game, because we don't always know what is going on for us internally. What better guide than your inner nutritionist, your gut feeling. Especially when eating trends and advice change as we learn more, it can seem like one minute so called expert advice says this and then they change their mind as something else is learned. That is the nature of progress. Tuning in and asking yourself, what's my gut feeling about foods and eating, what would benefit me self-care wise in this moment, what does my body want or need? I treat it as an experiment, I may try this or that for a while and see how my body responds and that can change from time to time too. My gut feeling, for me, is that in all likelihood what they say about red meat could well change, just as it did with margarine and butter. My body said it wanted butter, I gave it butter (in moderation), every time I tried to eat margarine it tasted plastic and false, it wasn't 'real' food and it tasted flat, with no vitality or life force. With red meat, my body likes it, guidelines tell us otherwise but my gut feeling for ME, is that my body wants it and does well on it. I have been vegetarian several times in my life but both of those times I was very ungrounded, so meat for me helps me ground. I send appreciation to the animals for that. However, as an animal lover I am open to being vegetarian at some point in the future if my gut feeling suggests so again.

## Energy testing

Some of us who are more sensitive may try holding foods by our solar plexus (see the Energy Hygiene chapter for more on the chakras), an energy centre which is just below the centre of the ribs. You may notice a feeling of stability and calm if a food is right for you, or an anxious fluttering if it isn't. It's thought that we can energetically sense from this centre whether the energy of something is right for us, maybe 'on the same wavelength' for us. Mindful Eating (see further on) can also help us to tune into food's 'goodness'. Slowing down our eating and paying attention to the texture, flavour and aroma of the food, truly taking time to appreciate it can alert us to whether we are eating vibrant and health giving food and how it feels in our body as we eat it, or is it processed, low vibrational 'draining' food? How does your body feel after eating it? Keeping a food journal can be a good way of monitoring links that we might not always notice. On a couple of occasions, I have had a seemingly healthy apple at the 'wrong' time (for me in the morning), and it has drained me. I felt worse after eating it than I did before. Going to see a trained kinesiologist may also be worth trying.

## Are you happy food?

Looking at the food on a deeper level and asking yourself, does it look vibrant, full of vitality? I ask myself does it look like 'happy' food, a vibrantly yellow glossy lemon that just looks plump, juicy and lush. As you are choosing food, think about what you are going to be putting in your body. With packaged, processed food, don't be fooled by the marketing either, it might not necessarily be true (think of the advert with the McDonalds burgers and how they are in reality for instance!). See if you get a vibe with the food.

## Coping with toxic invasions

A common sense guideline can also be 'if your grandmother wouldn't recognise the name on the ingredients label then don't buy it!' The more we mess about and change the way that food is formed, taking it away from it's natural structure, the more it 'denatures' as vitamins oxidise and fibre breaks down. My gut feeling since the butter/marge debate I had with myself thirty years ago, is do we really want to be putting foods in our body that are artificial, which the body doesn't recognise as food but could see as toxic? If this is so, doesn't the body then have to work harder to rid itself or detoxify from this? Pay attention to the things that you wonder about, it could be that your inner-nutritionist is trying to tell you something about the food that you eat. If we are trying to recover or rebalance from illness, it makes more sense to me, to put it under as little strain as possible. It could be that the body sees additives as a source of stress, if it perceives it as a toxic invasion. If we are in good health in all other ways it may be that this doesn't have much of an impact and we can cope with foods that are less than wholesome. But if coping with illness, especially chronic illness, or stress, my feelings tell me that I'm better off trying to eat as 'clean' as possible. On a couple of occasions, about to undergo an event with some stress, my intuition has guided me away from sugar as it has during the final stages of writing this book! I suspect to fine tune and help my body to function better during those times. Listen to your inner-nutritionist.

## Things change

Our life pathways take us this way and that. Things change as we grow and experience different cycles of the month and different life stages and as we age. For each new change it is worth asking ourselves 'is this right for me?' I can't say that anything is wrong for you, you may cope well with what I don't cope with and vice versa and guidelines are just that, guidelines. It was thought not so long back that a great way of getting your five a day was by having a smoothie if you weren't that keen on eating fruit. However now it's acknowledged that due to the fibre that is broken down, and the increased dose of sugar due to a higher amount of fruit, it is not necessarily the health kick that it was once believed to be.

If we were presented with the equivalent amount of whole fruit that goes into a smoothie we might not eat it all, certainly not in one sitting. It is a possible way to get your five a day if you aren't reaching that, but try having smoothies with higher vegetable content and one fruit, such as kale, spinach and pear - these can be really tasty. Generally, advice has gone back to just eat the apple whole as it is. However, pre-match if you are a sports person, or as I said, if you aren't getting your five a day, a small smoothie may well provide a quick burst of energy and much needed vitamins.

## Nutrition for smokers and drinkers

When I realised how smoking diminishes vitamin c, and if I cut myself it took a while to heal, I also began to take a high dose vitamin C tablet. I began to make my own food again after eating mainly processed food. I mindfully introduced foods such as ginger, garlic and onion to support my immune system. I knew I wasn't in the right place to give up smoking so did what I could to support my body whilst I did smoke, until a time came when I was more able to give up for good. This may also be wise for those who consume more than the average intake of alcohol, as that is said to deplete vitamins and minerals.

## Probiotics

Probiotics help to balance the friendly bacteria in our digestive system. They help maintain a balance in our gut health and are the 'good' bacteria in our stomachs. They are found in some foods. The gut feeling is something that has more recently come to light medically as awareness of what is called the gut brain axis connection is further understood. This highlights how the millions of neurons and neurotransmitters run between the gut and the brain. It was once thought that it was just the brain that produced the neurotransmitters, but is now seen that the gut also produces them. The environment of our gut and the role pre and probiotics play are now being seen as vital for our digestion as well as our mental health. And this bears up well and makes sense to me in my experience.

Back in 2000 I was going through a particularly stressful period, having moved house, and experienced an increase in the amount of sore throats I was getting. My diet, which had usually been good (80/20), had taken a downward spiral. For the first time in my life I was pretty much existing on processed foods. I look back and realise that is in part why I was so ill, but I was stuck. My inner-nutritionist urged me to take a multivitamin which contained a probiotic. Within a few weeks I felt significantly better than I had done for a while. I appreciate we are all different, and one size doesn't fit all, but my benefits from taking it lead me now to suggest to clients, if you can't do the five a day, at least take a multivitamin with a probiotic. They don't have to be very expensive.

Some say we need to buy the most expensive vitamins and minerals, etc., as they are more 'bio available' (better used) in the body, and this maybe true in some cases and for some people. However, I suspect, in part, it could be a selling point for companies to sell their own! I have benefited from some standard low-price vitamins and minerals as well as the opposite, finding that the vegetarian form of omega 3 from flaxseed didn't appear to be working as well as the omega 3 from fish. I appreciate the bioavailability argument but not in its entirety. It is finding out what works for us, so if you do suspect a deficiency, try experimenting.

## Nutrition for IBS

In more recent years one of my health challenges was that I was still suffering from irritable bowel. I'd overcome the worst of it, where I couldn't go out for 2-3 hours after I got up in the morning, so I would have to get up extra early. The thought of staying elsewhere had seemed impossible. It had a huge impact on my life as anyone who has suffered in similar ways will appreciate. This went on for years - when I had to go, I had to go. It started after taking an SSRI antidepressant which I had an adverse reaction to. Going back to the gut brain axis, I feel it disturbed that balance, along with antibiotics over the years. There are many things which can upset the good bacteria in the stomach, including sugar.

After seeing a dietician for IBS, she recommended a probiotic called Alflorex and the FODMAP diet. I cannot advocate trying pre and probiotics enough in the case of irritable bowel and mental health. The cheaper version had certainly helped on other levels, but what she had recommended was a lot more expensive - could it help with the IBS? It certainly did in my case prove to be worth it and helped me to fine tune the IBS and my digestive system better. I'd also recommend the FODMAP diet, which is difficult, but also helps to educate us which foods we may react to. Some of us have fermenting tummies! (especially likely if we consume excess alcohol and/ or are sugar addicts!).

Foods that are great for our gut health and feed our 'microbiome' are seeds, almonds, fermented foods such as sauerkraut and kimchi, and sprouting seeds such as red clover, broccoli and mung beans. Sour-dough bread makes great toast and for many is more digestible. Drinks such as kombucha and kefir, miso soup as well as peas, Brussels sprouts, olive oil, ginger and garlic may all be helpful. I particularly enjoyed Dr. Megan Rossi's book Eat Yourself Healthy as it was well explained, easy to follow and illustrated.

After struggling for so long, I marvel from time to time that I can now go out for a run within 30 minutes of getting up in the morning. Anyone who has suffered from IBS knows how disruptive it can be. Because the particular probiotic recommended is so expensive, (£25 for a month) I have since experimented with cheaper versions, some of which definitely didn't work as well, and others, now that I am more balanced, maintain me well. This is what I mean by experimenting.

## Exclusion diets and intolerances

The FODMAP diet excludes or limits various vegetables and fruits which are high in certain carbohydrates. These can ferment in the stomach causing bloating, wind, diarrhoea, pain and bowel changes. It has also become very popular for people to exclude refined sugar, wheat, gluten and dairy from their diet due to the affects that it may have on the body. For some these may cause bloating, possibly contributing to IBS, weight gain, candida and hormonal problems such as PCOS.

I was told about the possibility of wheat and dairy causing problems and it did strike a chord with me, with the IBS. However, I wasn't ready to go there and explore exclusion diets for ten years! I totally understand the fear that this can bring up in people. When I mention this possibility to clients, and ask whether they have investigated links, they look horrified at the thought of it. I reassure them that it is just something to think about and look into and it took me ten years! Plus, it may not even be their journey, as one size does not always fit all.

The thought of giving up those foods terrified and confused me, especially as there wasn't the range of the 'free-from' products that we enjoy today (though I have to say these are often processed and most of them, due to the list of ingredient s, I would prefer to do without anyway). However, what I'd been told about the exclusions, in terms of the health benefits, was reiterated by a friend on the holistic therapies course.

She'd felt so much better when she gave up wheat and dairy (and sugar) from her diet and others seemed to notice a benefit. The instructor from the gym that I was going to queried what I was eating (seemingly healthy diet, porridge for breakfast, homemade leek and potato soup for lunch) and why I wasn't losing weight. Again in the back of my mind my inner-nutritionist suggested that it might be that the inclusion of dairy in my diet causing me to hold onto my weight.

Finally, I came to a place where I wanted to lose weight and I decided to cut down and that really did help. I had to be in the right place to do it, but I noticed the weight dropping off as well as my skin getting clearer and less spots around my chin area. Not liking the substitutes I cut dairy out with few replacements, but if you do so make sure that you are getting enough calcium from green leafy vegetables or take a mineral supplement. Unfortunately I do find it difficult to maintain completely dairy free, but as I have experimented I've noticed that some forms of dairy I can tolerate better than others. Small amounts of lactose free milk I'm ok with, but cheese and normal milk in large quantities can set off my IBS again, (as can too much sugar). Cream and butter tend to be ok too - so if you decide to try eliminating, maybe see a dietician or a nutritionist for support and experiment and see.

It can quite often be the case for those that have excluded certain foods that they have had problems with in the past, commonly such as wheat and dairy, that on gradual reintroduction they are able to tolerate it better. It might be that the gut lining may have healed by having a break from it. Similarly, we may find that foods which have previously been OK with all our life, such as bananas, suddenly become an issue for us. I think as we enter different life stages and the balance of our hormone levels change, our metabolism changes, our digestion changes and this can also affect how we process and use food, perhaps its a bit like adult onset asthma or hayfever. Our attitude to foods and our appetites also change as we get older. We are in a constant state of flux, so just when we think we may have reached a point of balance, if we do have issues with food, it might be that we have to adapt things again.

## An attitude of observation

The Mindful /Intuitive eating approach that I adopt and teach is about retraining ourselves not to demonise foods. 'It's the dose that makes the poison' as Marc Jacobs says in his book about metabolism 'The Slow Down Diet'. My Nana used to say 'everything in moderation' which is a balancing attitude. Growing up, we were raised on grilled cooked breakfasts whereas I wanted cereal and toast like my friends! Over the years I've found that I do actually do better on a cooked breakfast or high protein. It leads me to wonder whether what we are brought up on does tend to suit us best.

When we cultivate a mindful approach to eating, we slow our eating right down. Try allowing yourself 10-20 seconds to consume each mouthful, making sure that you chew it well and notice what goes on as you do that. If you have ever savoured a food and focused solely on that food, excluding TV, reading, talking, etc., and noting the texture, flavour, how your body responds, etc., you have mindfully eaten it. It can occur quite spontaneously when we are on a slimming diet and may have a chocolate bar as a treat, letting the chocolate dissolve slowly on our tongue to eke it out. By really truly appreciating and making the most of it and wanting it to last a long time, we can slow our consumption down and enjoy it. If we were to do that with most of our eating, we can come to value and taste our food better , and cut back on overeating as we notice that we are actually full before we've finished what is on our plate.

Some, as they begin to eat more mindfully, notice that they are eating foods which they actually weren't too keen on! Again perhaps out of habit because we are told that they are good for us. Mindful eating is a relaxed state, which could mean that we begin to digest our food better too. How many of us wolf our food down, not giving it a second thought, then wonder where our attention actually was during the meal, or where the meal has gone?! I was a very fast eater before I started to eat mindfully. That can lead to overeating, so by its nature mindful eating can help us to stop overeating if we tend to do this. It helps us to put the brakes on. However, I do also joke that mindful eating led me to a croissant habit!

## Food as a cover

For years, every Sunday, it became a ritual for me to have croissants for breakfast. I particularly enjoyed the almond ones or the chocolate ones, often both. I would sit and eat them very slowly, savouring the crunch, enjoying the sweetness. If you remember a certain food advert that played in the UK where the delicious looking food was accompanied by a very sultry voice - that was my croissant experience! This went on for years! I would become anxious at the thought of not having the croissants. I wasn't addicted because I didn't want more and more of them but I came to realise that it was covering an issue.

This is another aspect of mindfulness. I sat with the process and allowed myself to feel all the feelings, breathing into them and relaxing and allowing whatever emerged to come up, not judging myself for it. You can try this too if you comfort eat, or are using food as a crutch.

What I came to realise was that I was using food as a boundary! I would get annoyed if anyone invaded that croissant boundary. What I was doing was creating 'me time'. Sunday morning and my croissants was my time for me. Because I wasn't creating those boundaries in other areas of my life, I was looking to the croissants to reinforce that. This was another reason that my Self-Care Sundays were born. Now I don't 'need' the croissant habit, but may still enjoy one every now and then. Are there any ways that you use food in order to cover up for deeper things that are going on for you? How could you care for yourself differently if so?

## Experimentation

In the spirit of experimentation, when my eye was drawn repeatedly to some cereal in the shop - a granola with plain chocolate - I thought I'd try it. I haven't had anything like that for years, not since I discovered I'd developed an addiction for a wholegrain cereal brand that I used to look forward to every morning. I started to notice that I would be rather panicky if I ran out of it (I think I'd possibly also given up smoking around that time). Then I realised how high the sugar was in it! I was astounded and stopped eating it.

Taking the cereal I'd brought to Aberystwyth to write, I had a bowl full of it for breakfast after my run. I ate more of it than I'd intended, it tasted processed and 'dead' and almost 'plasticky' like there was a false flavour to it. I probably only noticed this subtle undertone to the flavour because I am so used to eating freshly prepared food in the main now. Despite that, I wanted more of it. In the interests of experimentation I went with it and then had nerve pain in my legs, I felt like I wanted to go to sleep or to eat more, I was quite out of sorts. That experiment can do well to illustrate nutritional self-care. It's not about beating ourselves up and saying 'oh I shouldn't have done that, that's bad I'm terrible'. Rather, by cultivating an approach of observation, 'oh that's interesting that it has that effect on me'. We can focus on those ill effects and pay attention to them, in order to retrain ourself to not make those choices again. I repeatedly do with some things, but I have noticed that over the years that I have been doing this, my excesses are fading as I come more into balance. It has taken a long time and is not overnight by any means. Back and forth, back and forth!

Growing up, I was fortunate to be raised on a pretty healthy diet of home cooked meat and two veg and often fruit for pudding. We didn't have fatty rich sauces, the food was quite plain but not greatly appetising. We had fruit for break, and sometimes had some angel delight for pudding as a treat,. Sweets were once a week and a packet of biscuits between the family to last the week. Seeing my friends eating what they did, I used to feel quite envious. I did used to get upset when friends at school would have a taxi biscuit or a club for their break, or a packet of crisps. Things like that were a real treat and seemed far more fun than my apple. When I then became able to make my own choices, I wanted these 'exciting' things and therein my weight battles began.

## Sickly sweet

Over the years of being the kid in the sweet shop, having what I want, battling with weight, I have at last noticed that when I have more carbohydrates in my diet, too high a quantity, I have less of a desire for fresh fruit and vegetables. I wonder if this is so for some others. I've noticed that most people aren't getting their five a day and question in part whether the high levels of carbohydrate in the diet may almost dampen the body's desire for good wholesome food. High levels of sugar in itself can alter the palate so that when it is eliminated or reduced in the diet, foods start to taste more flavoursome.

High levels of sugar can also trigger the desire for more, more, more, particularly when combined with fat. The recommended daily amount of sugar for an adult is only 30g or 7 sugar cubes. It's not a lot at all considering how many processed foods contain sugar that we might not expect, such as pickles, and tomato sauce. The combination of fat and sugar is thought to override our satiation buttons.

Leptin is our satiety hormone which, when working efficiently, helps us to feel full so we stop eating. However, the combination of fat and sugar is thought to interfere with this process. I rarely have sugar during the day, partly for that reason, but will have it in cake or pudding in the evening. Just recently I've had another inner nudge to experiment with lowering sugar again and it's no surprise that I do feel so much better physically. Sugar can cause inflammation in the body, brain fog, it is highly addictive as it affects the same endocanniboid receptors in the brain as drugs do. I am well aware that when I have to much sugar I can feel mildly drunk on it (and start crying sometimes!), nor can I tolerate much alcohol.

## Slimming diets

No nutrition section would be complete without mention of slimming diets. I'm of the opinion that just as not one size fits all, it is about finding which slimming diet may help us best if we have weight issues. There are so many different approaches and beliefs and arguments to how we use and process food and probably just as many disagreements and contradictions and supporting beliefs. You know how you feel in yourself, tune in and as with experimentation, notice.

I lost about 3.5 stone intuitively eating. Having a good understanding of nutrition, my inner-nutritionist advised me of a diet plan, and it worked very well for me and at that point still got to eat cake at night! I got to a point where I became interested in other slimming plans, and tried those to see how I felt. I'd only ever followed Rosemary Conley's low fat diet, which I liked because I could still have sugar! I did well on that years ago, however, I didn't maintain it - as many of us don't.

I decided to then take the plunge and do the exclusion diet of low carb, no sugar, no dairy no wheat, no caffeine and it was hard but I did feel good for it. However, as with any of the stringent eating plans, they can be difficult to maintain. I also then noticed that I was binge eating, something that I'd never done before. At forty-two I thought I was developing an eating disorder. What I know now from my experimenting with various ways of eating is that deprivation doesn't work well for me, however I can do very well on fasting by itself. I enjoy that approach when I get an inner nudge to it as it feels like my body resets from it and there is some good evidence to suggest that we can do well.

I went on another work-based nutrition course during which we had to fill in a food journal which exacerbated my anxiety around food. We were encouraged to calorie count and use an app to do that which I enjoyed doing. I attained the lowest that I'd ever consciously been. But keeping it off was the problem, it was the yoyo approach, even though I was looking at the psychological issues where I could underneath. I think that is the large part of the journey of eating for many of us. Interestingly, my portion sizes had grown to a degree that they never had before, mainly with vegetables.

I tried another popular diet where you attend weekly to be weighed and otherwise don't have to weigh much food, but due to their freedom with certain carbs I started having those again - and also to see if it helped me sleep better, which it did. However, I also noticed that I did put weight back on and didn't feel great in myself physically, I was much more achy.

I began to realise that if someone invented a diet which helped to effectively maintain our weight they'd be very successful! Once we get our heads in the right place to lose weight and restrict our diets, we often can do it, the weight comes off but it's difficult to keep it off. This is where The Powers that Be decided I needed to read Beyond Chocolate, a fab book about ditching the diet. Combined with that, the Marc Jacobs Slow Down Diet Book and the Mindful Eating approach which I'd adapted, plus my own inner-nutrition diet, I looked to finding what was good for me. I also came across a book called Therapeutic Hunger.

I also came across a book about hunger, which encouraged us to just be and allow that hunger and be OK with it. In the past I had always panicked at the thought of it, my blood sugar wasn't particularly balanced and it was a vicious circle. The idea of the intuitive approach to eating says ditch the diets, eat what you want, but stop as soon as you are full works well for some as in that way we begin to self-regulate. However, recognising that this could be the case in my approach to teaching it, I suggest that your intuition may also point you towards slimming plans that work for you - and this may, over time, change too. Mindful eating had kept my weight stable for a while, however I then went into a place where I again realised that I didn't *want* to stop eating and was over-eating again…

If we look at it from an experimenting perspective, mindful eating helps us to keep tuning in and checking in to our body and listen to how it responds to what we put in there. Intuitive eating, in my definition, can point us towards what might be right for us in terms of our own eating plans.

So as some weight crept back on and whilst doing another nutrition course I returned to the tried and tested over the years calorie count. This approach I find quite grounding in helping me to take stock of what I am actually putting into my body, as well as helping to regulate portion size. So rather than cutting out various food groups, it is eating them in moderation - as the Eat Well plate suggests. I feel much better in myself and more level than I have for a while, so intuitively that's working for me right now.

## Five a day

I'd say that 95 % of my clients admit that they don't get their five a day, which may be a reflection of my client group, but nevertheless an interesting observation. We could be lacking something in the approach to encourage people to get more veg, vegetables, fruit and fibre. It's even being said that seven a day is more helpful in dietary terms, particularly if we are trying to include 30g of fibre in our diet to protect against bowel cancer and other illnesses.

Quite a substantial portion of vegetables or fruit is needed to obtain adequate nutrition from them; five portions of 90g servings which totals the recommended amount of 450g. If you look at a small bag of lettuce it is actually 90g. However, that can be eaten over the course of a few meals, like a side salad. So my motto about adding food to the diet, also comes with my mantra 'eat salad with everything'. It's said that the proportion of nutrients that we get from vegetables aren't as good today as in the past, as our soils are so depleted from intensive farming. This might be another reason to supplement your diet with vitamins, but you will know how you feel.

My suggestion, as well as eating salad with everything, would be to try eating your salad or veg first, before you eat the carbohydrate portion of the meal (if you do eat excessive carbs). I will even have salad leaves for breakfast. It sounds odd initially as here in the UK it isn't a classic breakfast food, but it can add some balance. For example if you fancy a grilled sausage and beans, putting it on a bed of rocket and spinach leaves tastes great. If you love pizza, have a large salad then eat a slice of pizza - you may even leave some! Bonus. I love a bacon butty, so I use a low GI bread or if I've made it, a homemade seeded bread with lettuce, tomato, onion, salad leaves and beetroot on it and it is delicious! The bacon is processed, but you can buy low salt bacon, or medallions, and even nitrite free bacon now. With all the other goodness, that's a good compromise on the classic bacon butty on white bread with lashings of butter. It forms a good example of the 80/20 rule.

Because I don't, as many people are also finding, do as well with bread, I am currently trying to make my own to see if that helps and at least I know that the ingredients are wholesome. I'm really enjoying my wholegrain seeded version and look forward to it. It's the same with cake. If I'm going to eat it, by making it, I've also burnt some calories doing so. It is amazing how many steps you can do in the kitchen alone; it really surprised me when I noticed this. Home made also lessens the impact on my body, there are no artificial ingredients or preservatives. I can even add more walnuts to the coffee cake for protein. Just tiny little adjustments can make for a marginally better balance and make us more aware of portion size (or eating mindfully when we are not!).

## Prioritise - get organised

To eat a wholesome diet we do need to be organised and that is part of the choice that we may make to eat more healthily. We may have to prioritise our lives and compromise our time in other ways. I think it sometimes depends how much of a problem we have with our health or digestion, as to the length we are prepared to go and the changes that we want to make.

My thinking is if all of this is too overwhelming, stressing about it will be counterproductive, so at least for now take a good multivitamin, power the vehicle properly. If you are forgetful, using one of those daily pill containers can help to remind you if you've taken one or not, or set a reminder on your phone.

## Good hydration

We are such a high percentage of water, our brain and body will function much better when there is petrol in our car! I'm not going to say much about hydration, but I know from my own perspective that drinking sufficient water helps skin health, stops headaches, helps my brain functioning keeping me more alert, plus keeps some weight off. How often do you mistake hunger for thirst? Having a glass of water when you feel hungry may stop you from snacking between meals. Another before or after a meal may aid digestion and making sure that over the course of the day you get the recommended 2-3 litres of water, may make quite a difference to your overall well-being. Alerts with reminders to drink can be added to your phone if you are prone to forgetting. Disliking water need not be a problem, it doesn't have to be plain water. I'd prefer not to have artificial additives so would avoid recommending those, but adding some plain fruit juice to flavour the water, or drinking a moderate amount of tea or coffee is still hydrating, just be mindful of the sugar in those. Herbal teas come in lots of different flavours too and can be a good replacement for conventional tea and coffee if you are also cutting down on caffeine.

## Caffeine

This can leave us feeling wired, on edge, restless and anxious as well as interfering with our blood sugar balance. Too much of it is an individual measure. I used to drink 12-14 cups of tea a day, a complete tea addict, and suffered from anxiety. I don't think it was the cause, but it exacerbated it and I did feel better for cutting it out completely for a number of years. That was quite scary for a tea addict, who not only derived comfort from a cuppa but also liked the social element of it as well. Tea can be so deeply embedded in the British psyche as a solve all. On reintroducing caffeine I limit it now to 4-5 cups a day. Again, this is a journey of trial, error and experimentation. If your inner-nutritionist suggests it may be a problem, try listening to that and see what your wisdom leads you to try.

Cut down on the caffeine, sugar, chocolate, alcohol, saturated fat, etc., if it hinders you. You probably know what will help and if you 'can't', treat yourself with compassion as well! Also, importantly, if you are iron deficient and suffer from anaemia, avoid drinking tea half an hour either side of a meal as it can interfere with the digestion of iron.

## Herbal supplements

I include this in the nutrition section because we can sometimes use herbs and spices in our foods as we cook. I particularly like chilli and ginger to help my metabolism, garlic and onions to support my immune system and turmeric to help with inflammation. Some of these can be bought as supplements. I, like many others, have really benefited from the latest' trend' of turmeric. With 'fibromyalgia' (CFS) aches and pains, I used to have a bath every evening to help with them, but since taking a turmeric, black pepper and ginger supplement I am saving on hot water. My aches and pains are substantially better and it is supposed to help with digestion too - however if I take too much I have funny dreams!

As mentioned previously I also take probiotics and I take other supplements such as omega 3 for the mind, evening primrose or starflower for my hormone balance, kelp for hair and nails and red clover blossom for hormone balance, as well as a range of multivitamins including calcium and magnesium, despite having a good diet.

I have never responded well to antidepressants or the herbal equivalents such as 5HTp or St Johns Wort, but I would suggest trying herbal supplements to see if they benefit you as some people have marvellous results from them. Bach flower remedies, such as the Rescue Remedy can also be good for helping people to calm anxiety. I would recommend that you do your research first or chat with a qualified herbalist, and if you are on on medication do speak to your pharmacist as some herbal remedies can interfere with medications.

## Rules around food

It is worth remembering that if we go the other way and have too many rules around eating healthy or 'pure' food and eating it may indicate an issue. Orthorexia, although not yet defined as an eating disorder, was coined by Dr Steven Bratman MD, and refers to the unhealthy obsession of eating pure, healthy food (whatever pure means to you). It can lead us to cutting out major food groups such as carbohydrates. I won't get into whether this is right or wrong, there's evidence of the benefits of the keto diet and veganism for instance, but rather it is our attitude towards this that can cause the problems. If there is an underlying issue with negative thoughts and feelings that are being covered up by the control of food, e.g. someone who is extremely healthy and couldn't eat a bar of standard chocolate (for example) without it causing them high anxiety. In cases such as this the person benefit from considering what is going on underneath these behaviours on an emotional level. A desire to convert or convince others that their way is the best way and the only way can indicate an issue. This isn't self-care; its a plaster, a crutch, a salve or a form of control.

# Chapter Sixteen

## Eco Therapy

### Nature therapy

Listening to the birds singing, feeling the earth beneath your feet, smelling the soil or the scent of the sea (or the smell of a river in flood as my partner pointed out to me); experiencing the exhilaration of water rushing by, feeling the sun on your skin, hearing the passage of the air or the wind rustling through the trees, these can all speak to our senses; grounding and soothing us. Even on a rough windy day, it can be exhilarating and there's much to be said for the saying 'blowing away the cobwebs'.

Connecting with nature, because we are a part of nature, is about coming home to ourselves and our true nature. Without the sun we would not survive, and as we have disconnected from nature, so can we disconnect from our being, our heart and our soul. It may also help with our physical fitness too, not only from an exercise perspective but people who get out into nature frequently seem to have fewer coughs and colds, as walking (exercise) stimulates the immune system and gets the circulation going. We may also benefit from the natural daylight, particularly in winter and especially if we suffer from seasonal affective disorder (SAD). It may help our vitamin D levels which are thought to be inadequate in the UK due to our lack of sunlight.

It is quite apt and intentional that I sat writing this section at Bwlch Nant yr Arian, a beautiful visitor centre in West Wales with forest walks and red kite feeding. The red kite is the national bird of Wales. The population of this bird of prey declined drastically and became extinct in England in the 1880's, and in Scotland too. In Wales there were only 12 pairs left.

At Bwlch, I experienced one of those glorious, profound magical events that is breathtaking, moving and humbling as well as inspiring! The Japanese call this Yūgen. During such moments with nature I feel like my ego has been stripped and the rawness of my spirit is revealed to allow something greater in, which is truly nourishing. However, we can't preempt these moments and demand them for self-care, they just happen when we are ready to receive. Mother nature knows best!

I'd gone along not really expecting anything more than an interesting experience. I decided it looked like a nice place to have a replenishing walk en route to Aberystwyth. As I walked along the path towards the hide, the sky was filled with a couple of hundred red kites. I looked up and tears suddenly streamed down my face. I hadn't expected that! I felt incredibly moved. I marvelled at nature and this gathering and how blessed we are to be able to interact or witness such amazing spectacles. There is a cleansing, clearing affect when we get out in nature.

Watching such a huge number of kites coming down to be fed and the thought that they could trust in humanity to come and feed, despite us nearly making them extinct, was quite thought provoking. I appreciate that them coming to feed is a self-fulfilling, conditioned reaction and they were unaware of our impact in that way on them - but can we really be sure of that? Who knows? The over-soul of a population is often thought, and experienced by some to link to a higher, connected level of consciousness.

However, I can certainly say for myself that my consciousness and awareness expanded. Sometimes this is known as Peak Experiences, as the psychologist Abraham Maslow described them. He said that they are 'rare, exciting, oceanic, deeply moving, exhilarating, elevating experiences that generate an advanced form of perceiving reality, and are even mystic and magical in their effect upon the experimenter'. (Maslow AH (1964) Religions, Values and Peak experiences. London: Penguin Books Limited) It is an ecstatic blissful feeling that is often experienced by those who love nature.

Many find this to be so as nature reflects something back to us, that when we pay attention, informs us of ourselves. Similarly, watching the starlings murmurate taught me about community and the nature of groups. We can project our consciousness onto these events in nature and by it's essence it can synchronistically provide a marvellous screen for this experience. It is no coincidence that nature can touch us on a deep nurturing level. It can be cathartic and transformative, a great teacher and speaks volumes when we quieten ourselves enough to hear both its call and its message for us as an individual.

After the experience, I reflected on the intensity of my feeling and what this said to me. It was touching my own depth of sadness from my own near extinction when I was repeatedly suicidal. I didn't think that I would live past twenty-five years old, but I had survived, as had the kites.

Another touching moment in nature may arrive by looking up at the stars in the sky and feeling humble in the great scheme of things, we are but a dot. Driving through the mountains has a similar impact on people, looking up at the vastness of them and feeling incredibly small. We may be struck by the way that the sunlight streams through the trees which touches our heart. Listening to a river in flood may feel exhilarating or the sharp sting of icy cold air on our cheeks on a cold winters day. There are many ways that nature can touch us and remind us of our vitality and fill us with hers.

We are such an integral part of nature and cutting ourselves off from the natural world cuts off a part of us too. We wouldn't survive without the sun, many of us respond and react to the seasons just as the plants do. We may hibernate in winter, and begin to bloom again when the spring comes and the sun shines, as we rouse ourselves and get out into the garden again.

## The elements

Working consciously with the elements can intensify our self-care. If I am feeling particularly heavy or sad vibrationally, and the weather is windy, I ask the wind to clear my energy field. Consciously absorbing the sun as it burns down upon us and asking for old energy that doesn't need to be with us anymore be burnt up and transmuted by the fire of the rays. Bathing in natural waters, embracing the coolness of the sea or a lake may help with the emotions, particularly depression, as well as physical aches and pains from the 'shock' of the cold water (try an ice shower or bath!). Feeling the soil beneath my feet or running through my hands as it helps to ground, centre and anchor me on this earth. These are all ways that we can link with nature's natural 'chargers'. Mostly we may do this unconsciously, but noticing it and mindfully doing so may bring forth greater insights and understandings of this marvellous world.

## Moon cycles and crystals

It seems relevant to mention here, in connection with nature are the cycles of the moon. It is well noted in the police force and A&E departments that there tends to be an influx of accidents and emotional flare ups on a full moon. Those of us that are sensitive may find that they have trouble sleeping or feel a bit emotionally wobbly or more intuitive around about this time and may also begin to notice a pattern with the new moon too.

Those who use crystals as part of self-care (see energy hygiene) may put them out, after cleansing, to charge with the energy of the full moon. It releases the old energy to make way for positive healing energy. The sun also charges crystals, but do be careful that they aren't left out too long as it can bleach them.

## Nature speaks to us, if we listen

At first we may not notice or be aware of the impact that nature has upon us and sometimes that will be stronger than others. But as we quieten ourselves, it can literally feel like receiving a blessing. The absorption of the peace that it brings to us, as the plants and trees vibrate at a slower rate to us energetically, can literally ground us and calm us right down.

When I started my conscious spiritual journey twenty years ago, an ash tree sprang up in the garden. It grew quickly, as we ourselves can! A few years later, during a bonfire in the garden a branch of the ash tree was burnt. I was mortified and very upset, but what it showed me was that it did literally spring from the 'ashes' as it regenerated. As I had. Like the Phoenix from the flame, nature reminds us that there are cycles of death and rebirth and sometimes something good can come out of adversity. A bit like composting - what we think is waste can break down and help something else to grow. What we think of as our waste can bear fruit in the future. As the saying goes, 'if life gives you lemons, make lemonade'.

## Nature bathing

Years ago I'd noticed that when I was out walking that I felt a soothing affect from walking under the trees and queried whether it was having some sort of positive effect on my energy field. Were the trees emitting something? It turns out so. They emit negative ions (like an ioniser, a salt lamp or like being by the sea) which has a positive effect on us. In Japan it's called Forest Bathing, or Shinrin Yoku and emerged in the 1980s as a national, natural way to wellbeing and they have gathered evidence for it's efficacy. As Dr Qing Ling says in the Art and Science of Forest Medicine ' when we are in the natural world we can begin to heal. Our nervous system can reset itself, our bodies and minds can go back to how they ought to be'.

It is subtle. Initially we may have to be in a quiet place to feel this. We may notice a different atmosphere when walking under different types of tree such as pine, or a variation in how we feel when we walk under our more native deciduous trees. We may just get a sense of feeling better and having let go of something or maybe something having opened up or cleared from us after a walk. It might be said that getting the circulation pumping and the air being forced through the lungs has quite an effect on us, which it does, but when we compare a treadmill walk or run, at the gym, there is something exponential that nature adds to the benefits of that exercise. Some people find it easier to communicate and talk to each other out in nature, and since lockdown it has sprung up as a viable way for counsellors to work with clients.

Running out in nature is an inspirational time for me and I am very fortunate to live near to two country parks. In the past, with agoraphobia, it had sometimes seemed like an effort to get outside, especially if it was raining. Learning to accept conditions as they are has been a learning curve. The different temperatures can be a teacher in themselves, how we respond and accept them when we mindfully stay present to the sensations. Feeling yourself soaked through, your feet squelchy with water, the rain running down your face then getting home and noticing that your face is glowing and that was a good 'facial' from nature, can allow us to really appreciate allowing and accepting things just as they are. Wishing that things are different won't change them, we can only be the change that we wish to see in the world ourselves!

## Our personal environment

While not eco-therapy in the true sense, as human beings we also need to take into account our own 'natural habitat'. Our home surroundings are important, whether consciously or subconsciously. Energetically sensitive people may find that their environment, whether that be at home or at work, can have quite an impact on them. If I go into a spiritual place where the energy is pure, it moves me to tears, sometimes even before I know the place has spiritual links. This I believe to be because the energy is freer flowing, clearer, thus more powerful - a bit like how a full river that is un-dammed rushes along. The energy pathways of the earth are known as ley lines, churches often said to be built on them. My first home was on one, there was a feeling of being at home and peace in that house, as if it looked after me - long before I understood energy. My second home wasn't, and I never felt settled there at all, quite the opposite. The home that I live in now is. Lying on the floor in the lounge is a lovely recharge point and great for yoga - and a place that my partner often falls asleep on if he's been out for a beer!

Conversely, places that have heavy negative energy can be challenging for those of us who are sensitive, It feels like wading through mud or getting stuck in quicksand. Have you ever noticed this yourself? See the Energy Hygiene section on house clearing to give your house an energetic spring clean.

The saying 'tidy house tidy mind', energetically, has some truth for me. If our minds are stuck or clogged with thoughts that are causing us to be stuck and we are focusing on other things, it stands to reason that our attention won't be on the house. This can have an affect both ways. We may not have the time that we would like to dedicate to clearing and tidying our houses. But it can become a vicious circle that we know we need to do but also drains us thinking about it.

Clutter, as well as the accumulation of dust and dirt can indicate an overly busy mind, perhaps ill health or simply a preference to do things other than housework. Not being able to let go of items, having lots of collections or a need to fill 'space' in a house, maybe a distraction to avoid looking at something going on emotionally. Living in an empty, tidier house, with less things in it could be quite uncomfortable for some. The minimalist space may be seen as empty with a lack of stimulation. However, where there is literally more energetic space to breathe and be, the energy and atmosphere can be calmer purely from an environmental 'busyness' point of view. Disarray and poor hygiene can be an indication of unfinished business.

## Home help

I received a lovely text from a client, who was overjoyed that she'd taken action on her desire to tidy the house and clear the clutter. She hadn't been motivated to do so for a while and had been struggling with this for some time. Having had various responsibilities in life, I did wonder and express whether it was 'her' time, to have some time. I enquired whether the possibility of having someone in to help would help her to 'get the ball rolling'. Sometimes when we have a little help, it can energise and inspire us. That input from another is literally energy coming in to our lives, which can give us a boost or a leg up. Her text informed me that she had decided to ask someone to give her a hand and things were underway. What a great feeling that is when that clutter gets shifted and things get organised.

## Make room for more

If my work isn't flowing and it is quiet or there is a gap in my client list, I will quite often look to see if there is anything that I need to attend to. I go to my self-care list of 'do I need different treatments or more treatments?', 'do I need to do admin', etc., 'do I just need time for myself?' or do I need to identify a block in the flow of energy? My intuition will sometimes 'draw' my attention to a drawer that has become rather disorganised and I find that almost as soon as I clear it, the bookings come in again. My sister finds the same.

# The keys to the 'place for everything and everything in its place'

This is pretty self-explanatory. On a practical note knowing where we have put something and trusting it is there saves time and energy. I was, and can be, by nature quite disorganised and I also have a memory that isn't the best, so I have had to put effort into consciously organising things . This is mindfulness in action, where we pay conscious attention to what we are doing in the moment. I have found that the effort has been worth it and that attending to returning items to their place, has saved me time over the years, now I have got into a better habit of putting things back where they belong. Apart from my keys, as I mentioned elsewhere! It's highly symbolic for me!

## The cycle of experience

If we recognise that we function well in a tidy house, because the energy is calmer and clearer, part of self-care may even be about clearing the clutter, doing the cleaning, clearing and tidying up because we know we feel better for it. A relaxed potter around the house, knowing how good I will feel for sitting down relaxing in a clear environment, is part of my self-care. When there are things 'to do' they are always there in the back of our minds, whether that is obvious to us or not. This consumes energy.

Being honest with ourselves about that can be a motivator to get things done, when we might not feel like taking out the rubbish or picking that sock up off the floor right now. An attitude of 'I'll do it later' can block the flow of energy and consume our own energy. As things are put on 'hold', it's like a road block or a dam; things build up. It creates a diversion which takes us the long way round and can become too much and feel overwhelming, rather than dealing with the small things in the here and now. It's the stitch in time approach.

An untidy house is a house full of unfinished business as well as blocked energy, in my experience. Recognising this was a key facet for me in recovering my energy from ME, learning to complete things. However, it did then give me so much energy and turn me into 'doing' mode. That is about finding a balance, a pendulum swings both ways before it reaches the place of balance.

Understanding how we respond when we act on things that need doing now, we may notice that it does make us feel good because that is an increase in energy. For example, whilst we are busy doing something we may also be needing to go to the toilet or needing a drink, but ignoring our needs (which become unmet needs). Putting it off is disrupting the cycle of experience. We put blocks in our own way. By acting on it and doing it, we often feel pleased with ourselves and a release of energy occurs - we have generated energy!

## A self-care goal

Knowing this and my past patterns of having many books that I am writing on the go and in progress led me to setting the goal to finish a book. If I can complete that cycle of experience it may also release the others. I particularly notice when clients come to me who are nurses, that they tell me that they don't get enough fluid because they don't have time to drink in their jobs. This I find ironic about the NHS (see Symbolism), because although the majority of staff do a great job, from the top the structure is not nurturing a culture of self-care for its staff. The organisation isn't encouraging its staff to take care of themselves, which can lead to ill health. Long hours and few breaks surely results in poor health, sickness and absences. I appreciate it isn't rocket science we're talking about, but it is nursing. Healer heal thyself!

What loose ends do you need to tie up and finish off? In your daily life what can you do in the moment to generate more energy for yourself?

## The right work environment

I'd heard from a few clients and a friend that Air b'n'b was a great way of finding affordable accommodation. I started to get Aberystwyth pangs as I do from time to time; it is my recharge place by the sea. I also thought it might be at last time to finish a book. My friend Julia, who is a VA, was redoing my website and commented how she'd benefited from reading it and I should write a book. I told her how I'd got many on the go, but thought OK time to give it another go. Come on God, let's do this!

The first house I clicked on said 'colourful' house (I'm a colour therapist) and it was run by someone called Helen (I tend to get on well with Helens) and she was a holistic therapist as well as having a cat. I took this all to be a good sign. It was the right environment for me, with a recharging sea view plus I was able to book in for a massage to top my battery levels up. I also found out that another lady rents the room who is writing a book and another lady who regularly rents is in printing. The only downside was that the gorgeous new kitten proved a positive distraction! I'll reframe that to a grateful break!

I don't think, as I have wondered from time to time, that I could have sat comfortably in one room in the Premier Inn and written for four days, much as I love that space with the direct sea view to stay in. I think the powers that be found me the ideal environment.

I told everyone that I was turning my phone off, so would be incommunicado apart from my partner, and my soul sis Yvonne, for whom I'd be contactable by email. All part of maintaining the boundaries of the right environment. When people are texting their energy does come in, which can be distracting. Although this is 'work' it still constitutes self-care, at work. The element of providing an environment that was conducive to doing the best job I can, is very much a self-care philosophy. Self-care isn't just about making our free time more 'power-ful', it is about caring for ourselves generally.

## Our energetic environment

Have you ever experienced that stillness of a power cut, where the electricity and all that background buzz in the air just goes? What a relief it is and perhaps why many of us like to go camping. If we are weakened in any way, such as illness, tiredness, etc., and perhaps generally too, it might be a consideration to turn off the Wifi at night or when not in use and only use the speaker phone on mobile phones and avoid using microwave ovens. Whilst they are all said to be perfectly safe, some of us are sensitive. There is some concern about the upcoming 5G, and the affects that this will have on our environment, wildlife and us; as it hasn't been introduced yet, the reality of this is an unknown.

Many of us who are in tune with energy may feel the effects of this and other wavelengths, and perhaps more so if we are depleted of our own energy. Being vital and well, 'having energy', can be seen and experienced as a form of protection. But not so if we are ill and depleted on some level. Shungite is a crystal and also Orgon pyramids, which are thought to help combat some of these wavelengths and give us some protection if you do feel vulnerable. My jury is out on these, but I certainly feel a benefit from using crystals to recharge my energy field.

It is my belief that this is progress, evolution. It is the world that we live in and wishing it was different will only drain us. Accepting the things that we can't control and changing the things that we can. Doing our best to live with it and to support ourselves in that process takes us forward. I might not like it, but worrying about it and fearing it will deplete me. I have noticed that the things that I used to try to avoid and felt could affect me now have less of an impact. As I have grown stronger, I have more resilience and have much more trust that my body can cope with environmental toxins and challenges. Fear of the changes will not help on top of the challenges themselves. Lack of faith in our own body's abilities to cope may be reframed into more strengthening thoughts and belief in ourselves, Or it may be that it is a call, that various issues of our wellbeing may need to be addressed and altered to support ourselves better.

## Gardening: self-care illustrated

Our garden can be a haven of energy for self-care that can help us to flourish too. So many of us gain a lot through our direct interaction with nature. It can be grounding, calming and satisfying, not to mention nourishing if we grow our own nutritious food. We can receive colour therapy from the flowers that grow and bloom and a great sense of satisfaction from our achievements. How idyllic! As we tend to and nourish our outer gardens, we can see how this is a good metaphor for our own self-care process. The more time and attention we put into our garden, the stronger it becomes and we bloom too.

The garden can also be a place of tranquility and relaxation, with natural birdsong, where we may also be able to meditate more effectively. Nature synergistically supports this process. Even if it isn't quiet, it can be good practise at accepting and screening out the various sounds. Our garden is bordered by a walkway where there are all sorts of conversations and noise is going on, that has sometimes raised my eyebrows! I found myself on a number of occasions missing the quietness of my previous garden. I realised that it makes for a more successful meditative process challenges the judgmental part of my nature!

Out in nature we aren't surrounded by the power and buzz of electricity (unless we are by a pylon). The energetic frequency and wavelengths of nature are said to be much slower, which can help us to slow down too. It may take time, years, for us to recognise our natural response to this, but as we tune in and practise this form of self-care the benefits can become more and more apparent.

Having a connection and bond with nature can yield much joy and vitality within us. It can help us to appreciate the cycles of life at a deeper level. Seeing that everything has a season can help us to accept our own comings and goings; we may be able to accept that it's OK to wind down and hibernate for the winter. We are connected to the earth, so it would be only natural to do this. We may also see that as plants die, that death is a stage of life, and with that endings are a natural process. And as seedlings grow we notice that with the beginnings we can experience new life, regrowth and flourishing that can occur as a result of that withdrawal of energy. Gardening allows us to embrace the exercise aspect of self-care, as we move around and bend down, it's often called 'the green gym; and I think of it as 'garden yoga' as I'm stretching.

Getting our hands into the soil and your feet in the earth can literally help us to ground. Seeing the garden blooming, nurturing and caring for the plants, looking at them up close and seeing them at a deep macro level develops our visual skills on a psychic level. It opens us up to seeing things that we hadn't seen or noticed before, it helps us to pay attention and focus. Interacting with the 'beasties' in the garden and marvelling at how they literally make the world go round, for example where would we be without the humble earth worm? It is a form of oneness, a feeling of interconnectivity, zoning out, meditating and when the sun beats down and I absorb those life giving rays, for me it's pretty close to paradise! It links me with my spirit and helps my heart to feel that joy, wonder, happiness and gratitude.

But what if we don't have green fingers? Or we don't have a garden. Accessing other gardens such as public ones can be equally as satisfying, as well as inspirational. If we aren't natural gardeners and don't know where to start, consider asking someone in to help who does know what they are doing. They may offer advice and teach you and from that you will grow too! If you have no garden space, plants in the home or planting some containers up may be an option.

As well as our own environment, self-care might also extend to our immediate local environment and might be something you could consider if you don't have a garden. We may gain a sense of satisfaction by going out on a litter pick (it can be addictive as well as satisfying!) and there is the social element too. Ask at your local park or beach, or contact organisations such as Keep Wales Tidy to see if there are any litter picks arranged in your area. They are glad of volunteers, and usually provide gloves, bags and litter picks. We may then foster a deeper sense of pride, care and appreciation for our local environment, which connects and benefits our growth too.

# Chapter Seventeen

## Animals & their rescue humans!

One of my favourite memes is of two dogs, behind bars, in a rescue shelter, one saying to the other, 'have you found your rescue human yet?' Never a truer word spoken in jest. Often we become rescuers because unconsciously that's what we really want ourselves. - to be rescued. We frequently do for others what we would like in our own lives, for instance we maybe loving because we didn't feel much love growing up and would like that. We may want to be rescued from the trials and tribulations, the trauma that we've suffered, the heartache, anything to take the pain away. And so we can't bear to see an animal or a person suffering. See the Healer Heal Thyself chapter.

Animals have a habit of showing up in our lives, and the 'right' animal, at the right time. I don't think that we always find them. Sometimes they can just turn up or perhaps our consciousness answers a call from them, if we do go looking and it all unfolds 'coincidentally'. I often wonder if animals are little angels in disguise as they can bring love, laughter, and soothing into our lives.

On a deeper level, they can also teach us a lot about ourselves. Sometimes they have their own journey of healing, due to their own trauma and resultant behaviours such as separation anxiety. Through us learning to understand them, they can teach us a lot. Even more so, when we bring the experience back to ourselves and ask ourselves what are they mirroring back or reflecting back to us.

A consistent stable source of love whilst growing up was from my interaction with cats, I think many people can identify with that animal constant. I loved animals. They didn't judge me and contact with them was grounding. I think many of us animal lovers feel that way about our animal companions. It can feel like they understand and accept us when no-one else does, not even ourselves. They show us their kindness in our moments of darkness. Although the responsibility of having an animal in your life if you are not well, can seem much greater, they can bring much healing to us, without us even realising until we look back on what we learnt from them being in our life.

Harriet and Hammond, who were brother and sister were the first cats that, as an adult, I had responsibility for. Animals just know! Harriet didn't leave my side when I was at my lowest points and sometimes became my sole reason for endeavouring to find a reason to want to stay in life. She did a very good job bless her, she was very much my soul kitty. Cats can teach us how to just be, what a joyful sound it is to hear a cats happy purr!

## Animals can give us a purpose

My goal had always been to get back to work, but I wasn't sure how to best help myself. Working on the premise that caring for my cat Harriet had helped me through some dark times, I decided to do something that I'd always wanted and give some other rescue animals a home. I wasn't going to have the small holding I always wanted, but I could rescue a few more cats and help to foster them. I also rescued a terrier called Tansy. I said to my mum one weekend when she came up to visit, I'd like to have some chickens. A week later I was out walking Tansy and there was a bedraggled malnourished chicken, who could hardly stand up. I had no idea where she'd come from, it was quite an isolated spot so I took her home, fed her up and after a while got her some friends - and she too found her purpose in life and crowed! Jemima was Jeremy!

My animal family motivated me to get up in the morning, if I couldn't always self-care for myself, I could care for them! Unfortunately, I went through times where I wasn't able to walk Tansy (and later Jake) because I struggled to go out of the house, especially alone. I was very hard on myself because of this ('negative self -talk', see Zap The Attitude for more) However, nowadays when I hear of others struggling with their own health yet wanting to give their animals or children the perfect life that they would like to, I feel more able to reassure them (and my old self back in time), that they still had love and food and company. 3/4 ain't a bad life! However, as we shall see later there can be a shadow side to that care.

## Poppy

As part of my plan to get back to work, I started volunteering for a local cat rescue. I fostered kittens and cats that were semi-feral. It was a lovely experience and something I could do without worrying about going out. Poppy was one of my foster kittens who I didn't want to re-home, she had to stay with me! She was a joy, such a happy little black and white cat, very dainty and pretty, and all the other animals loved her. She was one of those shining lights, gentle and radiant.

Some years later, Poppy became ill and wasn't getting better. I took her to the vets, she had a blood test and the vet told me that she had feline leukaemia. It wasn't something that she would recover from and nothing could be done for her. I was desperately upset and something within me stirred, a determination.

A thought occurred to me, what about alternatives? The vet agreed; I explored the options. I got books (this was before internet days). I went into overdrive, trying to find things that might help. I looked at nutrition and aromatherapy and found something called homeopathy. I located a local homeopath who agreed to see me; they can't charge for animals unless they are a vet themselves. Very kindly Dawn spent time with me trying to find a remedy. At this point Poppy had jaundice. As a homeopath, she prescribed a remedy and the jaundice went. The vet was surprised and pleased and since then uses some homeopathic and Bach flower remedies in his practise. The great thing about animals is that they don't understand the placebo effect! That also spoke volumes to me.

Dawn also gave me a remedy called Ignatia which was for grief when that time came, as it was likely that Poppy wouldn't be cured. I think the complementary approaches gave me some more time with her, that she might not have had, until she began to suffer. The awful decision to have her put to sleep was made. Bless her sweet little soul, she gave a great gift to me. After all the energy I had put into the research, obsessively, there was now a great void of time but also some relief from that intense care and worry. I took the homeopathic remedy Ignatia and it allowed me to grieve for her more easily. It wasn't as raw, it took the edge off so that I could feel the pain and let it flow through me. It helped me accept her death, allow the grief and appreciate her life.

Maybe it was a remedy that helped pave the way, maybe it was Poppy's gift to me, or maybe I'd started to hear or be more open to God's guidance - or all of these things combined. I realised that I would give my all to help the animals and other people, but I wasn't doing this for myself! Self-care was born.

## The shadow side of care

I've often thought that shops such as Pets at Home aren't totally for the animals, they exist and do so well because they fulfil a need in us, to take care of our animals. Going in and buying products can make us happy. In that we gain self-care and fulfilment too, because it does make us happy, but perhaps on a superficial level. *Sometimes it is our need to be needed.* However, being aware of that is crucial for not going into the shadow side of care, whereby people have too many animals, begin to collect them or rescue them, but can't provide them with a good standard of care. I noticed that I could quite easily verge on this myself, but circumstances illustrated that this wasn't a way forward. Animals in these situations can almost become like objects to be collected where they are filling a need in us.

The time I spent fostering cats and kittens for a cat charity where I also worked taught me a lot. I had multiple cats, several dogs, chickens, guinea pigs, rabbits, a goose and ducks. Caring for them gave me an awful lot, because their needs got me up in the morning when I wasn't able to do that for myself. However, I stood recently in Pets at Home and noticed a natural cat pheromone which is available in sprays or room diffusers. It is found to calm cats, it said, 'in multiple cat households'. Cats are quite solitary and independent; they like their own space. And it did strike me, are we putting our needs over the needs of cats by using products like that to try to get them to integrate? Is this about us or them?

I thought about the potential stress of introducing one cat to another and how that had been in the past. Was this product really developed as a result of our needs? If we were really considering the cats, maybe, knowing that they often prefer to be by themselves unless raised together, was this once again going back to the cat being an object? In cold, hard clinical terms, this isn't, however, as black and white as that. They are loved very much, but maybe loved for what they bring to *us*. I guess I can only own my own experience and say perhaps animals have been there to meet my needs, as well as striving to give them happy stable contented homes and in that it is a two way process. We meet their needs for food (I think we need to admit that with animals certainly a proportion of it is cupboard love, though certainly not all) and also the love that they give to us, helps us.

## Filling a void

This realisation came after I'd recently expressed my desire for us to get another kitten whilst our cat wasn't too old to find him irritating and was about the right age for another to be integrated. What I was fearful of was not having a cat. When an animal passes, it can be devastating, it can leave a void. And my partner had said himself, when his previous cat died, 'never again'; yet I came along with mine and they adore each other. For me, having a cat growing up filled a huge void of loneliness for me. I won't go into details, but there was a quality of being anchored by Cleo, and then Marco, Lilo and Sumo, yet when we hadn't had a cat for some years between Cleo and Marco my heart ached even more. There is something about the tactile feel of cats (or dogs or other animals) which enables many of us to be more present in life, it is soothing and calming and can lower blood pressure.

What I was bringing to our situation in the present, was the unconscious remembrance of that painful void, loneliness and emptiness that I'd felt as a child when I didn't have a cat in my life. When my partner said he didn't want another cat, nor did he think our cat would like another, I disagreed, but… read on. My concern was that as my cat and I had come as a pair, when our cat died, as he would eventually, he wouldn't want another. I couldn't contemplate the possibility of living without a furry friend in the house. However, what I realised was that with all the other tools of self-care that I have in my self-care tool-kit, such as allowing myself to feel my feelings and so on, that my need is not as great as it was. That was then, this is now.

## Letting go

When my dog Tansy died, then Jake died six months later, I consciously decided that I would carry on walking without them. By the time they passed I was going out and really enjoying the nourishing feel of nature at least once but often twice daily. So I carried on walking and it helped the grieving process to allow myself to feel their absence as nature soothed me. I can't count the number of times that I have cried tears around that valley as nature has dried them!

However, very shortly after Lionel came along, 'by chance' and found me when my friend said she couldn't re-home him due to a problem with his legs. I enjoyed the time and companionship that I had with him in the moment because as a breed Great Danes are renowned not to live long. When he died I didn't actually feel the need or want to have another dog at that time, because my priorities had changed. This surprised me! I didn't want the responsibility at that time, as I had started to go away and explore more by myself and although I could take a dog with me to do that, being tied to that wasn't quite right for me. So it's interesting how things change and how, as I have grown, my 'need' for my furry friends have lessened.

As I reflected on my partner not wanting another cat right now, I acknowledged my initial feeling of disappointment. However, as I sat with that, I realised that when I had looked for one, I hadn't been able to find or see a cat or kitten that pulled me to find out more. So I reasoned it probably wasn't the right time and was able to accept that.

## Recovery of 'being'

I realised that even if there was a void, when Pepper passed I could cope nowadays with that because I can allow the emotions to flow. It reminds me of how, during a conversation about our love of cats with my holistic therapies tutor, another Dawn, I said to her 'I don't know what I will do when Harriet (my soul kitty) passes' and quite rightly she said 'you'll grieve'. I did, and I got through it, better than I ever would imagined, but I always felt she would pass when she knew that I was going to be OK. So with that, I could let the thought of a kitten go, respecting my partners decision. The timing was either not right or we'd watch this space, but whatever unfolded, I could trust that I would and could be OK now.

## Animals as messengers

Over the years I came to realise that my interaction with nature and animals could reflect back messages to me, to deepen my understanding of where I am at in the world and within me. The symbolic meaning of animals or plants can be interesting to research, if they leap out at us. Many people are reassured by a robin, for example, feeling that it is a link with their loved ones in spirit. Doing so brings back the message to us, rather than asking another, and in that way can be empowering. The tradition of power animals or animal companions does that too. We may have always felt a pull towards a certain animal and understanding what that meaning is to us can be very informative.

For years as a child, I dreamt about riding around the housing estate I grew up on on a horse. During therapy, I ascertained that to me the horse symbolised my freedom. When I see horses cantering and galloping across open spaces, it brings tears to my eyes, possibly because I am yet unable to join them freely. Often we are locked in the prisons of our making, our consciousness can keep us stuck for years like quicksand!

The animals that we are drawn to and what they mean to us, such as cats and their independence and acceptance of that, can show us something about our own journey in life. There is no right or wrong in how we interpret the messages from animals and nature, only what is right for us - or right for another if that is different to our own meaning. We are all individual on different paths, so whilst a heron, to me, gives me a nudge towards focus and concentration and so meditation, to someone else it might symbolise go fishing! And it can also change or deepen in time, because today when I saw the heron, he spoke to me of stillness and out of the stillness. Likewise, a buzzard to me reminds me to have fun. The wren is my link with God and reassurance that I am on track. Observing animals in nature and how we perceive them, brings the message back to us, so the joy that the buzzards get when I watch them soaring on the thermals, calling to each other, reminds me to have fun!

If we feel that an animal, or maybe a plant, in nature is trying to tell us something, researching the 'symbolic meaning of...' in a search engine is really interesting. Similar to choosing a crystal in a shop, we may not know what it is or why we are drawn to it, but when we research it, find that there is something there which speaks to us in that moment.

## Equine Therapy

Despite the strong pull towards horses, growing up I wasn't able to fulfil that longing. As part of my healing journey, to get me out of the house as well as give me more exercise, I decided to take action and fulfil it. It happened quite by coincidence again, as 'the greater plan' often does. I was looking for straw to put in the hen house and drove onto a nearby livery yard. The girl there said that she didn't usually sell it, but would do this time. I saw the horses and thought to ask her if she did riding lessons. That was it, myself and a friend who had expressed an interest not so long back, booked in and off I went.

For anyone who loves horses, the smell of them and that relationship with such large creatures and the way that we interact is quite unique to that of our 'pets'. Therein started my love-fear relationship with them. Over the years I'd notice that just as I felt like I was beginning to relax and get my confidence, I'd get thrown off or something would happen and my confidence took momentous dives. I remember my friend saying 'you have to learn to stay on Emma' and she was right, in more ways than one. But I found it hard and I'd have gaps where it just wasn't in me to try, again.

Horses, being flight animals, were perhaps mirroring my own flight nature. They brought up such fear within me and I had a lot of it. Life has often cajoled me into getting back on though, just when I think the ride is over. So when I got that familiar pull again, I said to another Emma at the holiday cottages where I was staying, 'I wish I could get my confidence with horses'. She replied that really you needed a relationship with one horse in able to cultivate that. There was no way I could see that happening. I couldn't afford it.

Step aside for the greater plan, I love this journey. A couple of weeks later, I was driving along and approaching the stables. My intuition said 'go and see Helen'. I'd been working and just wanted to go home and have a piece of cake and a cup of tea, so I argued with it. 'Go and see Helen,' my intuition insisted again. No! I want cake! I argued like the petulant child I was! As well as the myriad of thoughts such as 'I haven't seen Helen for ages, maybe she won't want to see me,' etc., etc., my intuition insisted 'If you can see Helen, as you drive past, go in!' There was Helen, stood in plain view of the yard entrance. Gulp! OK.

She was as pleased to see me as I her and within a short time explained to me that 'it was funny that I was there'. I wasn't surprised, I am used to the way things unfold now regardless of arguing with it and wanting cake!. She told me that the girl who had had Thomas, who I had often ridden in the past, had just that day bought her own horse so couldn't keep him on loan. She was looking for someone that she knew that she could trust to keep him gently exercised in his retirement. Obviously meant to be. Then and therein started my journey with Thomas.

I soon realised I had to be more assertive. Just as Tansy my first dog was wily and wilful, so was Thom, and being assertive didn't come naturally to me - and that was what he was teaching me. Tansy had taught me so much, that I 'had to be in charge' but I wasn't that good at it and she could still wangle her way around me.

Animals, if we dedicate ourselves to that relationship with them, can push us out of our comfort zone and in that we grow with them. It isn't easy, it isn't pleasant but the rewards and what we learn can be tremendous. Thom was taking me up a level and so the journey began. I couldn't stand in my own power, with confidence, so I would go up to the field and Thom wouldn't budge, he'd stand there. After immense frustration of trying to ask him nicely, being grumpy with him and then crying, one of the girls from the yard came up and took his lead rope and walked as he followed obediently and I found a friend. I read the Tao of Equus by Linda Kohanov, so was aware that he was reflecting back the elements of me that were out of balance and did my best to work on that.

What I could do with Thom was limited in part due to his age but also due to where I was at, but we plodded along for a while, until riding him wasn't an option as he was losing condition, so he was turned out to graze. After riding another friends horse and having an accident, that was it for me again. And for a long time I didn't miss it.

## Equine facilitated therapy

Until I saw The Mustang. This film reignited my desire to have Equine Facilitated Therapy (EFT). I'd been curious how that would be, when I first heard of it some years prior. EFT is where a therapist works with you as you interact with horses. I had incorporated some of these aspects, as I said, after reading The Tao of Equus by Linda Kohanov, but I couldn't find or afford a therapist at the time and sometimes I feel that as part of our journey we need 'another'. A large part of self-care can be about allowing others in and letting them help us, but other times the timing isn't right.

Equine therapy can be about noticing our own energy and reactions, the way that we are and how that might impact in our interactions with the horse; what it brings up for us or what emerges. Rather than just 'blaming them' (if we were to) for not wanting to come with us when we try to lead them, we could look at what that is meaning for us in our lives, why have we attracted in such a horse etc., etc.

With Thom, it was apparent that I wasn't asserting myself, when he planted his feet in the ground, yet minutes later was confidently, in a no nonsense fashion being led off by my friend. Thom could read my fear and hesitation. Taking ownership of this is where we grow.

My sojourn into EFT, during the first couple of weeks, was grooming them and getting to know them a bit. I recognised that my fear of them rearing up and striking me was my past experiences with people (not horses) superimposed (or projected) onto the horses. It doesn't have to have been an experience that we have necessarily had with a horse, it can be experiences that we have in our lives with humans, but our subconscious projects itself into the situation and onto the horses. Observing and noticing this can then open things up. I think it is a gentler way of working than face to face therapies. The action of 'doing' around the horses takes some intensity out of the session, whilst also allowing me to work through some of my own fears, as well as some of my fear around horses.

Ironically, I hadn't really come to EFT for my horse fears, but hoped it may also be a facet and a plus that this could be worked through too. On week 3 I led one of the horses round the field. She didn't seem keen to come with me. Having had this issue with Thom being stubborn and his owner even saying he could be a bit of a bully (I attract them, to learn), I immediately thought it was about me needing to change my energy, my tone of voice, it was my responsibility. I wasn't assertive enough. This can certainly be so. However, I had also wondered, seeing her tucking into her hay net, whether she would have been far happier staying there.

When it came to leading the other horse, she came with me straight away, there was a willingness. The horse that I'd had difficulty leading was also reluctant to be led by the therapist. There was something going on with the horse. I felt relieved, it wasn't 'my fault', the onus wasn't on me! It wasn't all about ME, it was about her. That was a big lesson in not being overly responsible for other people, or 'horses' stuff. I saw that I had done this far too often and it was time to look at situations with an 'actually that's your stuff approach' too.

The next week as we discussed what had happened the previous week, it dawned on me what it was. Due to the sadness and fears of my childhood, I couldn't control anything. It was emotionally chaotic and emotional EQ wasn't understood. The one thing that I could control was by taking responsibility. If it was my fault, if I could change how I was and what I did, if I could people please, etc., then life might became more bearable. It was a survival strategy that many adopt. Consequently, if things weren't going right, I could either figure it was something that I needed to change about myself in the dynamic, and I took on the burden. And I repeated this in relationships.

I also realised that my fear of the horses kicking me were due to having been kicked by a person. My sense of powerlessness, with larger 'beings' (as horses are much bigger than we are), was brought home to me by my immediate ease with the little shetland Crystal. She is so small and cute, but in reality probably not as gentle as the others! I also realised, as Crystal got stuck into the food bag at every opportunity when the barn door was open, that was just like me and my inner child with cake!

And so that therapy continues for me, but our relationship with animals and how we are with them can form a large part of our self-care, with personal relationships as well as assisted therapy.

# Chapter Eighteen

## Exercise & Sleep

From one end of the spectrum to the other, but both serve each other well. A good night's sleep helps to repair and restore the body and exercise can help us to sleep. Both aspects are vital for self care so form a companionship within the same chapter!

## Exercise

This is one of my daily go-to's. I often say it's a miracle I can run as with chronic fatigue, taking a step feels difficult enough. The benefits of exercise are the endorphin release which gives us those feel good happy chemicals, better circulation, better bone health, weight loss or maintenance, better skin, more flexibility and so on. Suffice to say, moving the body, especially if we have a sedentary lifestyle, benefits so many of us. Finding the right exercise for you personally might be a creative process and a challenge.

With M.E. it seemed nigh on impossible. I remember one occasion where I couldn't understand how anyone had the energy to lift a spade in the garden! When someone has chronic fatigue, getting up to make a cup of tea can be incredibly exhausting and for others hard to believe, especially as people with this often look well. The body feels like it is made of lead, like having to drag a lead weight around. The thought of exercise can be the last thing we may envisage being able to do.

The green gym or the garden could be a good place to start to get more movement - even baking a cake in the kitchen instead of buying it, is getting some steps in. It's amazing how many steps I can take whilst cooking!

Walking is the tried and tested favourite for many, and is good for fat burning too when done at a pace of 'going to be late for work'. Combined with being out in nature for an energy hygiene clearing, it can be inspiring, stimulating and beautiful when we take the time to admire the view and soak it all up. See the Eco Therapy chapter.

Obtaining a GP referral from your doctor might be a good place to start if you haven't done exercise for a while and have ill health. Physical trainers can then assess you and your needs. They may advise exercises such as nordic walking or a local gym class which does circuit training. There's also the social aspects of that too where working in a group can provide distraction from our struggles as well as social support and encouragement for each other.

I'm not trained in exercise therapy, so can only really talk about my own journey with exercise and what has helped me since I began to use it for self-care. My own history of exercise was checkered. Up until eleven years old, I used to play tennis regularly at a local club. Gym was more difficult as my balance and therefore confidence wasn't great. I didn't find that running was something I was good at. This wasn't just a mental wall, but something physical related to chronic fatigue possibly, which I experienced as difficult and which has now fortunately changed. I think it was an indicator that something was out of balance even in childhood, as is sometimes said to be the case with fibromyalgia (walking up stairs and hills had always been very difficult too). So perhaps if you do struggle with exercise, it could be a health imbalance and might be worth getting it checked out.

After twelve years old, I had various experiences - cross country running at school was an opportunity to go for a cigarette, as I'd started smoking then! In the sixth form at school I went rowing, the circuit training associated with that was difficult and I went back to running again. I joined a gym in my late teens but found it so boring, and not enjoyable at all. Despite wanting to do it for the benefits, like many of us I guess I didn't want to put the effort in. This is another reason why I say it is a miracle that I now enjoy exercise and appreciate the benefits of it, so please take heart if you struggle too, it might be just finding the way that is right for you.

It is a great part of my life that helps my energy to flow, stimulates my immune system, clears my head and I receive inspiration and 'mind processing' time. It is meditative for me, and I experience many other benefits; if I don't exercise I begin to notice that my body and mind don't feel as good. But it wasn't quite as simple as knowing that I 'had' to exercise and I'd benefit and then 'doing' it.

## Resistance

For the average relatively fit person it may also not be as appealing either and a real struggle feeling like you 'should' exercise. We may be aware of the benefits of exercise, that good muscle tone helps to support the skeleton and bones thereby powering us. It promotes good circulation, speeds up metabolism and helps the lungs and heart health. It also has mental health benefits with all of those endorphins rushing round, which might mean help with anxiety and relaxation, as well as better sleep. What a great advertisement for self-care. Yet how resistant we may often be about doing it.

I knew that I 'should' try to exercise more, as many of us do. I tried to fathom out what I could do that I felt able to do and that I would enjoy. I decided to do something that I'd always wanted to do since I was younger and learn to ride. I found a local riding stable and soon realised that it was a good form of exercise, you don't just 'sit' on a horse, Being around them and taking care of them is also a good form of exercise too. Because I was so passionate about it, and my desire so strong, it gave me the motivation and perhaps the distraction too, to push me through my fatigue. Gradually my energy levels seemed to increase slightly, though they still went up and down.

I was given a yoga DVD to review for an online store and really enjoyed learning from that. Over the years since I ventured out more, I have gone along to various teachers for sessions. DVDs or online classes can be a good option for trying exercise at home if you aren't too keen on the social elements of groups.

I'd started to go for more walks again, with the dogs and tried to do some gardening but this was a struggle at times. But gradually and over time, as the homeopathic remedies, vitamins and other self-care strategies kicked in, I began to find my levels of energy got to a point where I started to wonder about going to a gym.

I couldn't fathom how though, because at that point I was still having trouble driving over the first big roundabout that led to town and there was no way I would have the confidence to walk into a huge gym full of people, even at a quiet time. My anxiety was too great. Instead, heaven sent, I was driving past a local community centre not too far from where I lived and noticed a sign saying 'gym'.

As I drove past I thought, I could drive there, and if it was under £17 a month I could stretch to that. It was £17 a month, it was a tiny gym, rarely used and very quiet. I was often the only person in there and I loved it! I built myself up gradually and did well, I wasn't even finding it boring like I used to when I was younger. I allowed myself to feel the physical, mental and emotional benefits.

## Flight not fight

One day whilst out for a walk with my ex-partner our conversation was quite negative and my irritation began to verge on an argument, which I knew was something triggered more from my past than the present. The fight or flight response kicked in and I thought about all the times in the past that I wished I could run away from situations and realised that I could mindfully use that energy literally and take flight. So I said 'I'll see you at home' and ran off! I got a bit further and carried on and thought to myself 'I can do this!' It was a real moment of achievement.

The next morning I woke early at 6am. I thought 'what on earth am I waking up at this time for?' and my Inner PT said 'take Lionel (our dog) for a walk and do a walk, run, walk, run'. So I did. I listened to my body and my inner PT about how far to go and Lionel came with me. I came back home feeling again like I'd really achieved something. Given the fatigue that I had felt, it was amazing. I wasn't so bothered or self-conscious about what I looked like. The walk, run, walk, runs soon turned into run, run, run and I built up to about twelve miles or so. I soon realised that all of the times during my childhood when I wanted to run away from home (and it was frequent) were stored tension in my body, and now I could actively and consciously let it out in a literal 'flight' mode, which is anxiety depletion management!

I never fancied the idea of entering any races, I just enjoyed being out in the beautiful surrounding countryside and being able to actually run. I joke that technically it's a miracle as I was so ill at one point, I felt like I should really be running with a couch strapped to my arse! I'd also been swimming regularly at the local pool and was really enjoying the feeling of my body working again. I realised that I had become obsessed with exercise as many people do, enjoying the endorphin rush, and I found it very hard to have days of rest. I was buzzing!

After a number of years I felt like I had begun to outrun all or certainly most of the flight that I had stored in me from my past. I reasoned then that I would tune into my Inner PT and listen to what my body wanted to do. Now I go on short runs, I don't watch the time, I just enjoy my connection with nature as I run and frequently receive Divine inspiration and gain new understandings as I do so. I run mindfully. I tune in to how my body feels. If I notice any sensations of e.g. knee pain, I observe it witness it and it often passes through (and I go for osteopathy if it doesn't). I notice my breath and the different stages of that, as it changes when I run. I stay present to my energy levels and how they change according to the incline or decline and observe the feeling of the different muscles as I run. I hear the birds magical songs and appreciate and have gratitude for their music, the sound of the river and the variety of sound it makes as the levels change. The jay that perches on the railing and its colours. It is a beautiful way to start the day.

Just this year I was very ill with a chest infection and it marked a good break of some months from exercise. I was a little nervous about putting on weight and becoming depressed again. However I was walking to work and over to the park, just not running and swimming. I made a decision to stop swimming for now and cut back on the runs to just half an hour mainly, three or four times a week, sometimes with some yoga at home afterwards. I don't go if my body doesn't really want to and sometimes I might have a lie in instead. It is nice to have that balanced approach to it now instead of the all out frenzy! How do you feel about exercise? Is there is form of exercise you could try?

## Sleep better naturally

I often say when I'm running workshops and courses that we teach what we need to learn and although I tend to fall asleep quickly myself, mostly, I've had my ups and downs with sleep over the years. In the past I've been awake for many hours through the long night before the days of the internet and all night TV. The main ones for me, still, are not going to bed earlier and waking up through the night, but overall my quality of sleep is a lot better until the new moon! I find that I am often more energised in the evenings during winter and inclined to go to bed later and more tired at night in the summer! As many people who are sensitive do, I find that the clocks changing and artificial lighting can really send me off kilter.

Having much better levels of energy nowadays, it has also surprised me how little sleep I do need when I am functioning 'well'. I think that in large part this is down to a healthier, balanced diet, so above all I advocate that for sleep, as well as the holistic therapies.

Insomnia is Latin for 'no sleep'. Seven hours is a general recommended amount of sleep to get per night, but we are all different. I often wonder whether by trusting that on some level your body knows best and has decided that you only need five hours sleep and that's right for you, it can take some of the 'I haven't had eight hours' sleep' anxiety away, which is tiring in itself. The amount of sleep that we need can change with age. As we get older, we may need less.

As part of our SC plan, getting a good night's sleep can help with our mind, body and spirit. It is like switching the computer off, or pressing our reset button so that we can update - the work can be done in the background. I've noticed for myself, that by eliminating certain anxieties about sleep, such as clock-watching and timing the amount of sleep I've had, I don't tire myself out all the more by worrying about it. I trust that my body knows what it needs for me. However, I know that isn't true for all as there are countless reasons why we aren't sleeping and it can be extremely frustrating waking up feeling like you haven't had enough sleep when you have a full day to get through ahead. So here are some self-care suggestions for getting a better night's sleep.

## Setting the scene for sleep

Use your bedroom only for quiet, relaxing, peaceful activities, so that your brain starts to link relaxation with this particular room and forms an association with switching off. Avoid playing games, using the computer, listening to upbeat music or other activities which you find stimulating and which may wake you up. I can't take a phone or i-pad up to the bedroom otherwise I get distracted and start Googling - then that's it, I'm wide awake again!

Minimise electrical equipment in the room such as TVs, computers and equipment such as phones with Wifi, that still run throughout the night. This is not only from the perspective of noise but also because they emit positive ions which are thought to contribute to energetic stress. To reverse this generally, as our homes are full of electrical equipment, an air ioniser or Himalayan salt lamp emits negative ions which mix with the air. This is then thought to be more easily absorbed by the body, reducing stress hormones and helping us to feel more refreshed. Having some plants in your bedroom, may help as they give out oxygen at night which is great for us. Plants that also purify and take toxic household chemicals from the air may also help. Spider plants are good at this, or mother in law's tongue is quite robust if you aren't great at taking care of plants.

Crystals including rose quartz, selenite, amethyst, blue lace agate and celestite may all help to set a gentle tone in the room and can help with sleep. They radiate such beautiful calm energy, as well as having beautiful colours. Of which, the colour scheme in your room is also important. Traditionally, yellow is said to be too stimulating for sleep so try to avoid this colour if it does affect you in this way. Pastel colours, or shades of blue and lilac may promote relaxation and calm, helping you to drift off. Make sure that the lighting in the bedroom is restful and relaxing as you are winding down and getting ready for bed – rather than stark, bright and too wakeful. Do your curtains let too much light through on summer mornings? You may benefit from buying a black-out blind if so.

How is your bedding and nightwear? Is it comfortable? Do you need to buy anything new? Egyptian cotton is supposed to be the most comfortable, but my partner finds it's too cold - everyone is different. Synthetic fabrics for nightwear may not agree with you if you get too hot at night, so check fabric labels; cotton lets the skin breathe. On an energetic and hygiene level, washing your bedding weekly may help even on a psychological level, as many of us do 'feel' better with freshly washed bedding. Check that you don't have any allergies to washing powder or fabric conditioner. How's the temperature of the room – if it's too hot, turn the heating off earlier or turn the radiator down in your bedroom, and get a fan in summer if you can bear the noise. If it's too cold get a higher tog duvet or a blanket for one side of the bed if you and your partner's thermostats are different. A different tog duvet for summer and winter may help. You may even want to try a weighted blanket as the heaviness is said to help soothe some people.

Does your mattress need changing? Having one that is as good quality as possible is a good investment for self-care considering the amount of time we spend in bed. Being comfortably supported may help with physical pain, if this is keeping you awake. If you are stressed during the day, is it because you have an uncomfortable mattress which means you can't sleep? Consequently due to lack of sleep, you might not handle stress as well as you may do, had you had a good night's sleep. This could be a vicious circle. Your mattress also may need turning, don't forget to do that regularly too. Is your mattress big enough? You will sleep better if you have more room! Also consider the pillows you are using. Do you need a neck pillow (I found that very uncomfortable!) or a thinner pillow?

De-cluttering can improve the energy of the room. Ask an energy therapist, such as a Feng Shui expert, to help you to arrange your furniture for maximum energy flow. I slept in a room recently where the chi was completely wrong for sleep, it felt so odd! Considering removing pets from the bedroom if they disturb you. Much as we may enjoy their company, you may notice quite a difference if you have more space for yourself.

Play relaxing, soothing music. There are many apps and videos on youtube available through the internet which have calming music, hypnotherapy sequences, or meditations which can help you to sleep.

Many people find the aroma of the essential oil lavender helps them to drop off. You can buy a lavender sleep pillow, or put a few drops of lavender essential oil on your pillow, be careful that it doesn't stain the fabric; do a test first. After two weeks, stop using the lavender oil for a few weeks to give your body a break from it. Alternate instead with chamomile, petitgrain or neroli. An electronic aromatherapy diffuser can be used to emit the scents before bedtime so the room smells calming as you enter it. If insomnia is linked with depression, bergamot may be a good choice of essential oil and is lovely blended with ylang ylang which may also help with sleep. Benzoin may help you to relax if you are a worrier. Sandalwood, patchouli and marjoram also have a sedative effect. There are also sleep sprays available from chemist and health shops. Do check with an aromatherapist or your pharmacist if you are taking medication, are pregnant or have health conditions.

## Throughout the day

Don't lie in on a Sunday if you have trouble sleeping on a Sunday night before work and feel tired on a Monday morning. Monitor your caffeine and sugar intake. Watch out for it in tea, coffee, coke and Pepsi and energy drinks such as Red Bull, Monster energy drinks, (hot) chocolate, guarana and proplus. Other stimulating drinks such as peppermint tea and ginger tea may also affect the sensitive, causing wakefulness.

Is your diet balanced? If not, taking a simple multivitamin may help. I find if I am on a low carbohydrate diet I have too much energy and can't relax, but too much and I'm sluggish. Going to see a nutritionist may help to identify a lack of any of the minerals and vitamins in your diet which may help us to relax and promote sleep, especially so if you have restless legs too. The mineral magnesium can help with sleep and relaxation and having an epsom salt bath before bedtime can induce drowsiness. Check with your GP / pharmacist that the restless legs are not a side-effect of any medication you are taking or the symptom of an underlying condition. If none of the above work, try a massage blend which you can rub into your legs each night which may help to soothe them. Exercise and stretching exercises, cutting out or down on smoking, and drinking may help.

If your sleep is interrupted by thoughts, perhaps they intrude because they need to be given time and your attention? Perhaps you need some quiet time. Switch off the TV or radio and allow yourself some peace to just notice your thoughts and pay attention to yourself. This can be in the form of just peace and quiet whilst going about your daily chores or by consciously sitting down and allowing yourself to think during the day. Also allow yourself to sit and feel, don't deny your feelings as they may want to be noticed too.

Meditation may also help you to relax if you are finding that stress is a cause of you not sleeping. Meditation helps to calm and quieten the chatter of the monkey-mind! Guided meditation MP3s are readily available over the internet or you may find classes locally; mindfulness classes are also worth looking into. Yoga is a relaxing form of stretching exercises which usually conclude with a meditation. This may help you to chill out in the evening in preparation for sleep. Holistic Therapies such as reflexology, Reiki and massage may help. So many people comment that they sleep better after treatments, however there are some who find them energising and if that is the case having treatments first thing in the morning may counter balance that.

Exercising more to tire yourself out physically may also reduce any stress that is causing lack of sleep. Becoming tired through exercise may help if you have a sedentary lifestyle. Exercise in a way that appeals to you and that you enjoy, hiking, dancing, Zumba, gardening, horse-riding, swimming, the gym, martial arts, wall-climbing – there's lots of ways to get fitter. Three hours a week can make a difference. If you have any medical conditions, ask your GP or see a personal trainer for advice on the best way to incorporate exercise into your lifestyle with your health condition in mind.

## Preparing for bed

Get into a routine. Try setting a reasonable time to go to bed and stick to it in order to allow your body to begin to feel tired; the time is the goal. Notice if playing on the computer, or electronic games past a certain time wakes you up again and if so, avoid them. For example have a cut off time of 9pm if you go to bed at 10pm, to allow you an hour for your body to settle and relax rather than racing round a track as this may be too exciting and overstimulating!

Cultivate self-discipline; this is my down fall. Know your 'go-past-it time', i.e. the time that if you don't go to bed, you begin to wake up again. Learn to go to bed when tired, listen to your body – pay it some attention and respect. We wouldn't expect a car to keep going on empty.

Chamomile tea and night time teas are very relaxing and drinking a cup of this in the evening may help. Chamomile tea is easily available from supermarkets now. The Pukka brand make a nighttime tea from lavender, oat flower, limeflower and valerian which is pleasant. Warm milk, Horlicks or hot chocolate are often useful to help people get to sleep.

Don't sleep during the day; if you are in the habit of doing so, try and do something active during your low, sleepy points such as going for a walk or doing some housework.

Have a warm bath as mentioned previously. The heat will begin to relax your muscles and if you have a proprietary or home-made bath blend such as lavender and chamomile essential oils, this may deepen your relaxation further as well as using magnesium flakes or Epsom salts. If using these and aromatherapy oils in the bath you will need to stay in the water for about twenty minutes in order for them to soak into the skin. You can also buy ready made bath sleep blends – just don't fall asleep in the bath!

Are you too hungry to sleep? Have something light to eat before bed, like a banana or a small bowl of porridge. Bananas, milk and porridge contains tryptophan which is a pre-cursor to serotonin, which may well help you to sleep. Other foods include cottage cheese, chicken, rice, pasta, potatoes and sea food. Magnesium rich food such as green leafy vegetables or a supplement, or bath, may also help. Having too much sugar may waken you up, as sugar is a stimulant.

Some people may find that spicy, garlic and fatty foods interfere with sleep; cheese, bacon, cured meat and chocolate contain tyrosine which is stimulating. Alcohol, contrary to belief, may disturb sleep; it may help you fall asleep but the quality of sleep when under the influence is poorer as it stops people from reaching the deeper stages of sleep.

Give up smoking – nicotine is a stimulant. It's a fallacy that it helps people to relax; having a cigarette stops the onset of the withdrawal symptoms which cause people to think that they are relaxing, when really they are not withdrawing. Nicotine can make it more difficult to fall asleep, and can even cause nightmares.

If you are snoring and wake yourself – or your partner – up, check for factors such as being overweight, smoking or drinking which can contribute. Try over the counter remedies, or chat to your GP especially if you are exhausted the next day or your partner notices you stop breathing briefly as this could be an underlying condition. If your partner snores, try some ear plugs.

If you are teeth grinding, mention it to your dentist who may fit a guard or prescribe muscle relaxants, as well as focusing on reducing smoking, alcohol and other factors which may exacerbate it. Try having a holistic facial or facial massage to help to relieve the jaw area and any tension there.

## Once in bed

Sex might be what the doctor ordered; an orgasm will release endorphins which are probably one of the best sleep remedies, helping you to relax and release muscle tension as well.

Have you got 'to-do' lists going through your mind? Reach across for your pen and paper and make a note – hopefully this will stop it from going round and round in your mind. Many people find that reading helps them to relax and unwind and they fall asleep with the book open, but avoid page-turners!

Listen to a guided meditation or relaxing music to help you unwind, or go through a series of exercises such as tensing each muscle in turn and then relaxing it. Inhale your lavender or sleep spray and just let go and fall back into sleep.

If you need to get up to go to the toilet, try to have low level lighting as bright lights may wake you up.

Don't clock watch if you are in the habit of worrying the next day that you only got 'x' hours of sleep last night; cover the clock over or hide it. Clock watching can exacerbate worry which can contribute to you feeling even more tired the next day. When you don't know how many hours sleep you had last night, you may be less inclined to focus on it, and just get on with the day.

## Still not sleeping?

Get up! If you are uncomfortable and have been lying there for ¾ hour or longer get up (don't have a cup of tea!) and do something relaxing such as reading, listening to relaxing music or doing relaxation exercises or meditation until you feel tired, then go back to bed and try again. By getting up, instead of lying there the theory is that we won't associate the bedroom with wakefulness by lying in bed awake. The bed is a place to sleep, not lie awake.

Book in for treatments – one of the positive side-effects of holistic therapies that people often comment on is that they may go for regular aromatherapy massage, reflexology or Reiki, to address pain for instance, but then also find that they are sleeping better too. Insomnia can be targeted directly through these treatments and often people will say that on the day of the treatment they have had the best night's sleep that they've had for ages!

Get to the root cause – check in with your GP who may look for physical reasons why you are not sleeping or psychological reasons. In this instance counselling may be of benefit. Over the counter remedies such as Nytol, Bach Flower Sleep Rescue, Kalms for sleep or melatonin may be of benefit. Boots and Holland & Barrett have good ranges.

Try learning Reiki or other relaxing therapies. Many people who are Reiki trained find that they sleep better and that if they can't, that doing a self-treatment helps them to go back to sleep. On waking early in the morning I give myself a Reiki treatment while I am lying there, so I can quite happily lie in bed for hours just relaxing.

I come back to my biggest finding for me with lack of sleep, is to not to lose sleep over it. When we are fighting it, wishing that we were asleep as we lie there tossing and turning and thinking that we only have two hours left before the alarm goes off and why aren't we going back to sleep etc., we are using energy up but also not accepting reality. As I've made peace with not sleeping, by doing Reiki, it has become much easier. And, as I've also said, it is only from my own perspective that this helps me, as always it is a unique journey and finding out what works and what doesn't work for you may be a process of experimentation.

If you have had difficulty sleeping for a while, it would be advisable to consult your GP. Also try keeping a sleep diary to help you to identify patterns in your sleep, such as how long it takes to get to sleep, what times you wake up and how you feel the next day.

# Chapter Nineteen

## Energy Hygiene

Have you ever walked into a room and suddenly felt a heavy atmosphere or vibe? Do you feel depleted around certain people? Do you feel emotional or churned up inside after being with someone? You may have noticed someone who looks like they have a black cloud over them, there is a clogged appearance around them, a ground down 'air' about them. It's something that we may not always see literally in the physical, but we get a sense of.

Have you ever had that feeling that someone has dumped their baggage on you if not intentionally certainly not responsibly. Maybe they've said something a bit off. A so-called joke which doesn't seem funny or there's been a dig. You may suddenly feel weighted down, heavy, emotional, upset perhaps with an intensity that shocks or surprises you given what has occurred. That's what we as holistic therapists call negative energy (sometimes known as Wetiko)

If you are working as a helping professional or therapist with people who have a lot of deep emotional trauma, or who are ill or if you are around people who are especially negative, energy hygiene, taking care of your energy is a must. We can't take on new energy if we are weighed down with our own or another's baggage - we cannot energetically carry it all! Some form of energy hygiene practise ideally needs to be carried out after every client, or incident, and certainly once a day (in the shower is often a good time for many).

Our energy bodies (the aura or energy field that surrounds us), are like a sponge when we have a high degree of openness and empathy. If we have similar unresolved issues that mirror what is happening for another, we can consequently take that energy on board. They leave feeling great and we feel out of balance! For example, if working with individuals who have suffered from sexual abuse, this may not have happened to you, but the psychological effects of the trauma might be similar to issues that you yourself have experienced. This leads me back to my firm belief about personal development, personal development, personal development, so that our old issues are not triggered by others and we can be a clearer channel.

Looking after your energy body or energy field is like taking a psychic shower. Over time that which we sponge and absorb from others can filter down and affect us on the mental, emotional and physical levels. The overwhelmed, hopeless, bogged down feeling which can precede burnout leaves us less resilient and on some levels more open and vulnerable to incoming energy. Irritation and anger can follow and tension that is then held in the body as a result can bring on the muscular aches and pains on a physical level. Due to the increase in stress, it may follow that we become more susceptible to viruses such as colds and flu... and so on. This might be helped, or minimised, by taking good care of your energy.

## Identify your open doorway!

First and foremost comes identifying within ourselves why we may be absorbing and sponging energy. Asking ourselves why we are taking something on or why we are open in the first place may help us not to. This can explored during supervision sessions, peer supervision or counselling. Does this person remind you of someone from your past? Sitting in contemplation may help. I have a long-term client who I am very fond of, but sometimes feel very drained after working with. I realised that they remind me of the nice side of someone I didn't get on well in the past, so it was triggering and bringing something up for me and my trigger to over-give of myself and my energy. Understanding why our door has been left open to someone can allow us to consciously shut or open it when needs be.

## Techniques

Some of the energy clearing techniques involve mental visualisations. Don't worry if you aren't a visual person, it may still work for you. You can try tuning in on a feeling level or a knowing level that 'it is done'. Setting the intention is the most powerful aspect of this work, because energy follows intention and intention is a transformative energy. Unless you are extremely sensitive you may not necessarily notice a difference each and every time. How you are and how you feel over time and with repeated practise (if it appeals to you) might be the best illustration of whether it is working or not. It is also worth remembering that not every method will appeal or work for everyone, but do experiment and see which suits you best.

## Prevention is the best cure - meditation and mindfulness

It is worth mentioning this to begin with, because ultimately it's better for us if we don't have to deal with clearing an overload of energy. Many of us believe that meditation strengthens and energises our energy fields. We boost ourselves up by plugging in and recharging with meditation.

Naturally helping us to clear by resetting our breath and activating our sympathetic nervous system to calm and de-stress us, this is importantly a preventative technique too. If we are strong and resilient energetically, we are more likely to let things 'bounce off us', we can 'shrug them off' more easily, rather than them sitting on or in us. A strong bouncy energy field is a bit like a good waterproof coat where the rain just drips off; so does 'negative' energy when we maintain a good energy field.

## Therapy space and house cleansing

My therapy room and home contain crystals which help cleanse and clear the energy of the room, such as citrine and selenite. Smudging your room and your energy field (and house) can help to move old, stuck or toxic energy away and clear it. Californian white sage or the British equivalent Mugwort is are piquant fortifying herbs that when lit give off a pungent smoke that many people appreciate the aroma of. I also offer to smudge the auras of some clients who seem particularly weighed down with heavy energy. Smudging with sage is similar to incense which can be used too. As the smoke is wafted (sometimes with a smudging feather) around the room or the person, the intention is set that it helps to clear and cleanse the energy. A door or window is left open to allow the old energy to leave.

Using Reiki symbols and visualising a silver violet flame to clear the room are other methods. In my mind's eye, I see a silver violet flame burning up and clearing the negative energy. I will also sometimes sit and send Reiki to the place where I am working if that feels right (but never to people without their permission). Some people sprinkle salt around the boundaries of their rooms or homes as a form of cleansing and protection. Having salt lamps or an ioniser in the room where you are working can also help to clear the energy.

A mirror can be used to deflect energy back out, e.g. a nightclub or pub opposite may be sending out heavy energy which doesn't belong in your room, so positioning the mirror can redirect it back out. Other people ask for help from the angels, Archangel Michael being a particular favourite with therapists. Direct to Source, 'Dear God please remove the negative energy in myself and this room. Thank you. Amen' is also another option. There is always Feng Shui, I don't work with this myself, as I generally have a feel or sense of the flow, but a qualified practitioner or even someone who is just interested maybe able to shed some light on the energy flow in your room. I notice in my therapy room there are possible areas of stagnation, so being mindful of those and paying particular attention to them can keep the energy from building up. It's a bit like a river or a pond where you see the bits collecting in one corner and things don't seem to be moving there so it all collects and needs dredging or clearing!

## Carrying crystals

Many therapists have crystals in their rooms to help to absorb some of the energy and/or carry them on their person. There is a joke amongst female therapists about the clatter of stones falling to the ground at night! If clothes don't have pockets, many of us will tuck a crystal tumble stone in our bras and often forget when removing clothes, as the crystal clatters to the floor as a reminder that its there!

Citrine is particularly good as it is self-cleansing ( I must admit I still do cleanse them, there's lot of information online about how to do that). Labradorite is a special favourite of mine, as I do find that it helps to stop energy being leached from my energy field. I always think of it being good for nurses too, as they are working with people who are in need of so much energy, so carrying a piece of that round with you may help to keep your energy for yourself. Black tourmaline is another of my heavy-weight favourites, for really helping me to ground when I'm up against really tough energy. Obsidian, may help us to understand why we are absorbing the energy in the first place by shining a light on our own shadow which leaves us open. Black kyanite may help with a detox, as may black moonstone.

The old favourite, rose quartz, helps with heart healing as well. We are always at our strongest when we can stay centred in the heart and come from a place of love. Many therapists also like amethyst for protecting their energy field and rooms. A grounding crystal such as red jasper may help us to maintain stability and balance. If we aren't grounded with good roots then we are more likely to come unstuck and be buffeted by the strong winds of energy coming at us.

## Therapy Routines

There are many routines and methods on the internet that you can find. Mine consist of a before, during and after routine that is ingrained in my practise. It's worth noting that as our routines become automatic, we still need to be present in order to pay attention to what we are doing, as this focuses the clearing work.

Before treatments I check into myself and notice whether I am grounded or not. If not, I feel the connection or link with my feet on the ground. This feels like a tingly magnetic pull from my feet. Some people see tree roots growing out of their feet into the ground below, to ground themselves. Others may protect themselves with a bubble of white or blue light, see more details later.

During a treatment, as I'm working, I imagine holes in my feet which are the minor chakras, or energy centres, on the feet. I set the intention that any negativity that doesn't need to be there is draining out through my feet into the earth below to be transmuted and recycled by the earth. As I am working, I sometimes feel energy coming off a person that comes through me. I then breath out consciously, seeing that energy as dark energy which I am blowing into a visualisation of a silver violet flame. This sets the intention that it is burning up and transmuting the negative energy into neutral energy, for recycling.

After the treatment has finished, I go and wash my hands and imagine that the connection is then cut between myself and the other person and that any negative energy is just flowing down the drain to be transmuted by Mother Earth. I will often go to the toilet for a pee, to mindfully release from my physical body any negativity I may have taken on.

## Other forms of clearing and strengthening

Over the years I have used various chakra (energy centre) clearing techniques which I will explain more about in a bit. I found that I had good results over a few years using a little known practise called connective therapy. This works with the aura specifically and holes, rips and tears in our energy fields. Think about the phrase 'torn off a strip; and how we may feel violated; this could be an energy field tear.

At the beginning of my journey I had aura photos taken and there were obvious holes, or black clouds initially. These were due to depression. Also at the time I was smoking cannabis to see if it would help with the depression and anxiety. Certain practises weaken or strengthen our energy fields, such as mental emotional and physical abuse, drugs, negative self-talk and thoughts, poor nutrition, etc. As I progressed with the daily meditation using the connective therapy technique, as well as Reiki and others, my aura became stronger and fluffier. It is good to have the visual pictorial evidence of the progress I made with my energy field.

You may also want to make yourself a room spray for clearing. Using spring water, holy water or sea water and a few drops of aromatherapy oil such as juniper, grapefruit, frankincense and lavender, a teaspoon or so of vodka to dissolve the essential oil in first and shake it all up. Put it into a spray bottle. You may want to put some crystals in the water, such as rose quartz, amethyst, clear quartz or obsidian and as my friend mentioned recently, sitting the mixture overnight in the full moon may intensify it.

## Exercise

Walking home from work, out in the open, also helps me to shed absorbed energy. If I am feeling particularly clogged, going out for a run gets the circulation going which is a clearing affect for me - noticing how the sweat pushes out of every pore any negativity. This can be quite cleansing and cathartic. And a shower afterwards to wash it all away!

Swimming I have also found particularly effective due to the motion of the body, as well as the clearing and cleansing effect of the water. This is something that can be done if a client has been particularly upset and it has triggered something for us too. If that is so, sitting and allowing ourselves to feel that emotion and releasing it in the form of tears, is also a good cleansing balm for the flow of our energy. If we can't go for a swim, another good method is a salt water bath, either dead sea or Himalayan salts, or even Epsom salts if you suffer from aches and pains as well. A walk by the sea consciously inhaling the salt air into the lungs for a clear out can work wonders.

## Essential oils

Juniper berry is an essential oil I always associate with clearing and detox. It can be good for clearing energy debris by combing it through the aura. A few drops can be dissolved in 20ml full fat milk and added to a bath (with grapefruit and fennel). Be mindful of using if you have kidney problems, are going out in the sun or have sensitive skin, it may tingle! Frankincense, as an essential oil, combed through the aura is also thought to protect and strengthen the aura in advance of a troubled client, or for the troubled client if they so wish and you are trained to use the oils.

## Showers, breath work and chakra work

A white light shower is a mental visualisation of seeing white light pouring down into my aura and through the top of my head into my body, much like a shower. I intend that the energy is cleared as it runs into the earth to be transmuted. Combining this with an inhalation of white light which fills my body and clears it, I then breathe out black smoke and see it leaving the body. I do this until I am only breathing out white light again. A similar method for Reiki practitioners is hatsu rei ho, and the dry bathing or brushing off routine, as well as a Reiki shower.

Working with the chakras, the energy centres around the body which take in and give out energy is a similar way to the white light shower. In this visualisation I see the energy centres being cleared and cleansed too. It maybe that the chakras which should open and close naturally in response to life, may be stuck open, leaving us feeling vulnerable or stuck. If they are stuck closed it may leave us feeling blocked. We often have a sense that our energy is not flowing.

My initial thought about the chakras was 'a load of tosh' - until I experienced them first hand after a period of regular meditation, when my root chakra started buzzing!! As I've journeyed along this path my experiences have proved invaluable for accepting some of the theories about the things that we can't see!

If you aren't familiar with working with the energy centres, an example you may probably relate to is the sensation when our heart chakra opens spontaneously. For example when we see someone in trouble or in pain, the empathy that we feel for them can coincide with a sensation that our heart is swelling or bubbling over with love and something is leaving us. To me, that is healing energy, coming straight from the heart. This literally goes out or towards that person. That is our heart chakra opening. Other times it might be that someone is telling us something seemingly quite upsetting or troublesome, yet we feel nothing, our heart chakra is closed. That could be because we are burnt out and have nothing left to give - or it might be that the person is spinning us a yarn for attention!

# The chakras

For those who are not familiar with the chakras, here is some basic information. The Sanskrit name chakras means 'wheels of light', which I always thought rather airy fairy. Far more understandable for us unfamiliar, ignorant Westerners(!) to call them energy centres. In simple terms, they are energy centres that give out or take in energy. I was taught intuitively during meditation, that they work like transformers do in an electrical substation, that they step down or step up the energy that they take in or send out.

To demonstrate this, I intuited very early on that one of my life 'missions' or ways of working, was to take spiritual information and ground it into more realistic, comprehensible ways so that people could more easily relate to it via their own experiences. To do that requires me taking ideas from higher consciousness (crown chakra or higher), filtering them through this energy (chakra) system, processing it and grounding that information so that the message is translated or communicated at a common sense level. A good example of when the lower chakras, for instance, are blocked is when someone who is highly spiritual isn't able to convey with common sense what they are experiencing in the spiritual realms on an earthly level. So the chakras work like processors and filters.

The chakras lie in the energy field above the physical body. The are seven major chakras which follow the path of the spine, from the perineum to the crown of the head. They all have corresponding body parts which they link to. To illustrate, we will use the example of the second chakra or the sacral, which in the physical body links to the womb for instance. The chakras link also to emotional elements, such as in the case of the sacral chakra valuing ourselves, or on a mental level it can correlate with thoughts of worthlessness, as well as spiritual elements and abilities such as 'clear feeling - clairsentience', or connection to the energy of the Divine Feminine.

Understanding the chakras can help with our personal development, and in this way is a great navigator for deepening our conscious awareness. There are major chakras as mentioned and also lots of minor chakras, such as those on the hands feet and shoulders.

**The Major Chakras**
- *Root or base chakra* at the base of the spine or perineum - associated with the colour red - relating to our security and survival, flight or fight, anger, energy, ability to be grounded in spiritual terms and our bowels, genitals and blood physically.

- *Sacral chakra*, located  two finger widths below the belly button - orange in colour - links to valuing ourselves and others, our feelings and emotions generally, our sense of worth, our bladder and womb and spiritually clairsentience (clear feeling), as well as empathy.

- *Solar plexus chakra* lies just below the ribs in the centre - its colour is yellow and it's our power centre. When this chakra is functioning well we can stand in our own sense of personal power, we have found our niche in the world and can empower others. Linked in the physical to our digestive processes and our gut feelings in the spiritual.

- *Heart chakra* is in the centre of the chest near to the level of the heart - green in colour - the fulcrum of the chakra system, where heaven meets earth (as above so below) and we come to a place of being balanced and working from the heart. Most people are often top or bottom heavy, so clearing from either end can help us to gain more balance. The heart chakra relates to the physical heart and lungs, a deep sense of unconditional love and connectedness to all there is, a connection with nature and healing abilities in the spiritual.

- *Throat chakra* at the base of the throat - electric blue in colour, our throat and thyroid are linked with this chakra as well as our ears and nose. The throat chakra is our voice, how we communicate with the world and our ability to be truthful with ourselves and others, as well as clairaudience (clear hearing) on a spiritual level and also channelling of spiritual information.

- *Third eye chakra* in the centre of the forehead just above the eyebrows - purple/indigo in colour - the third eye connects with the pineal gland in the brain and our eyes. It is what we see within and without. On a spiritual level it connects with clairvoyance or clear seeing and also with our personal development what we see within ourselves or what may be reflected in another, it is our ability to look within.

- *Crown chakra* situated at the top of the head - violet or white - the crown chakra links to our spiritual awareness, consciousness, faith and beliefs, whatever they may be (a scientist for instance, science is their faith)it links to the pituitary gland in the brain which is the 'control centre' for the hormones, of which the chakra system is very closely linked! Hence why as we are clearing we can experience turbulence!

As I have said, knowing where our physical blockages are can highlight some of the links to the mental and emotional or spiritual issues that may also benefit from being addressed, by understanding the chakras further. It also lends itself well to symbolism and 'body talk' where the body can be helping us to understand ourselves at a deeper level from the symptoms that we present with.

## Nature clearing

As mentioned in the section about nature therapy, walking under the trees which give off negative ions can help to clear our aura in a positive way. Feeling my feet on the earth and letting the wind or the air 'blow away the cobwebs' is a daily ritual for me. Either running or walking, especially by water can help to soothe our emotional body, or even better by the sea with the salt air to clear negativity.

## Clothing & Colour

Mindfully using colour, especially when associated with any blocks we may have with the chakras, can help. Black is absorbent, so might not be great for therapists, although it does also provide an 'invisible cloak'; those who don't want much attention and to fade into the shadows may chose to wear black. Dark blue, navy and indigo are good colours to wear for pain relief as they are anti-inflammatory colours (think of blue plasters) and staying quite grounded. White is reflective so may reflect the light back to someone. Yellow is a stimulating colour which brings joy and happiness and orange can be good for working with emotions and emotional release. Red is energising, but may also be inflammatory as in the case of anger or a red rag to a bull, and also on a physical level, whilst violet is a calming, spiritual colour.

## Bubbles

Some therapists will imagine or visualise themselves being surrounded in a bubble of white or blue light. The idea behind this is to protect ourselves from invasion in the first place. Visualising and surrounding yourself in an egg shape of white light or blue light with the intention that you will be protected from negative or harmful energies or just setting that intention and knowing it is done, may be useful for you. A concept that works better for me is the idea that if I am vital and well, my aura is a natural egg shape and that it will be fluffy and full (like a good hearty cloud in the sky, as opposed to a wispy one!). So seeing myself with the dense energetic field, either white or blue, works better for me.

Another method, similar to the white light shower above, is seeing the energy coming in through the top of the head (the crown chakra) and as it fills our body, it starts to come out of the pores of our skin and forms an egg shaped bubble around us, which protects us. We can even visualise a 'repellent' intention, much like waterproofing repels rain, setting the intention that our energy field will have a repellent effect from negative and energy that we don't need just 'washes over us' and flows away.

## Cords

Invasion or draining of energy maybe also be via what are known as energy cords. These are links that are thrown off subconsciously or consciously when others see us as a good supply of energy. An indication that someone has attached to us is a change in our thoughts or behaviour, we may be thinking about the person frequently. Cord cutting is a mental visualisation of seeing yourself and any cords which are attached to you being cut. Some people ask Archangel Michael for help with this process. Using the crystal obsidian can help to cut these cords.

However, most importantly I feel is the consideration on the psychological level of doing shadow work or counselling (see that section). Often it is our unconscious stuff, which has left the door open, or there is some mirroring occurring which attracts various people towards us. I ultimately think 90% of the time these experiences are leading us to a deeper understanding of what is our stuff, so taking responsibility for our own projections, rather than blaming others, is always a healthful way to go! We can blame someone for coming in to steal from our house, but if we keep leaving the front door open, where does the ultimate responsibility lie?

## Nutrition

From a nutritional point of view, there are various herbs that we can take, either as supplements or that can be included in recipes that I feel help clear my energy fields as well as being tasty and nutritious. I've been drinking a lemon and root ginger, with cyder vinegar in sparkling water drink for some weeks now and noticed the refreshing energy clearing me as a I drink it (that came as an after-feeling, I just fancied it and hadn't intended it for that purpose). I also have on my desk at work a dropper bottle with organic rose water essence in which I have a few drops of every now and then notice an internal energetic clearing. Rose always symbolises unconditional love to me.

I also think garlic (think about the old vampire tales!) rosemary, lemongrass and chilli are also cleansing for the energy field. Detox teas and other formulas such as the herb Pau- D'arco may help us to work from the inside out and may be worth a try, as this is another approach, if you are feeling that something is stuck. On that level a parasite cleanse might be worth investigating, or a homeopathic cleanse, especially for times when it may be that we feel that others are 'feeding' off our energy. Sometimes the outer can mirror the inner (the macrocosm and the microcosm). Often it is the case that we are susceptible on a few levels. If there are parasites in our gut, possible if you have animals, clearing them may help to restore the vital balance of flora in our systems.

## Energy that's been dumped

With regards to energy that has been dumped on you from another, such as in the case of a toxic childhood, or an abusive relationship, as your awareness grows of what was their stuff and not your responsibility, you can forcefully ask that any energy that is not yours leave right now. Send it away 'for recycling', or ask God, the light or the angels to take it away. Smudging yourself as you get rid of that toxic energy and repeating 'this is not mine, it was yours' may help you to separate from that energy and help to strengthen your boundaries and heal any holes in your aura or energy field. If you continue to think about it, it is likely resonating or attached to some of your own stuff, so contemplating that or working it through with a friend or counsellor can help to release it.

## Treatments

Self help may involve asking for help from another. As part of my physical as well as energy clearing routine, I have treatments weekly from another therapist, see that section. This keeps a flow going of clearing my own stuck energy and also that of others which may still be sitting on or in me. Treatments such as Reiki, Angelic Energy Therapy, Diamond Energy Therapy, acupuncture, homeopathy, Spiritual Energy Therapy can all work specifically at helping you to clear your energy field, and are not limited to those mentioned. Physical therapies from another therapist, such as massage, with use of oils can also help you to keep clearing. It is an ongoing process.

## Worse case scenario

If heavy weight energy is projected at you, it can cause quite a lot of damage to your energy field, as I have mentioned previously. It can sit like a layer on top of people and can be absorbed (such as in the case of negative thoughts and programming, we are told we are a 'bad person' and start believing it and telling ourselves that). This can and does cause real problems if it is severe and not dealt with. It is not dissimilar to the concept of 'possession', as if a part of that person has been taken on board, the echoes or energy of which are within us, and we need to get rid. This is something that you may either ask your Helping spirits, God or Jesus to help you to clear (ask for inspiration on what to do) or to go and see an experienced therapist. This may be an Energy Therapist, counsellor, trans-personal or Jungian psychologist who is open to energy or a spiritual life coach.

## The learning curve of self-care

Over the years of trying the bubbles and cord techniques, at various intervals, I've not found those methods to be effective for me. I needed to understand about psychological boundaries and saying no, about not over-giving and sometimes taking too much responsibility for other people's stuff. For example by thinking that they might just be in a bad mood, and it's not necessarily something I've done, it closes that energetic doorway - whereas when I have thought I've done something, I've left myself open to see or feel their energy, and made it about me. So, that's taught me, for my journey. I often find that if something doesn't work for me it is because I am going to learn more for myself and often because I am sharing with others too. So if some of these methods don't work for you, try something else, we are all different and that learning will be sure to teach you something.

# Chapter Twenty

## Further Ways

Let's look at some more practical ideas for self-care. Remember self-care is not a stick to beat yourself with! Rather, it is trying to find things that nourish us, that make our heart and soul sing. The things that fill us up, or on a more subtle sustainable level drip feed us with energy, so the cup stays more full.

## Drip feeders and Quick Tips

### Basic Hygiene

To those who do this as a matter of course, it may seem an odd self-care tip, or indeed a given. However, with mental health problems in particular, some people find it very difficult to find the motivation or have the inclination to even wash their face or brush their teeth, let alone have a shower and wash their hair. This lack of self-care can be because the person has lost care. They may no longer care about themselves and what happens to them. Things may feel so futile, just getting through the day and making it to the next is a big achievement in itself.

It may be that if they are not fully grounded in their body and have cut off feelings, they don't even notice the feeling of needing to wash, and can't appreciate the difference when they do. Sometimes, on a day like that, the achievement of washing your face and brushing your teeth is huge, so remember when you do to give yourself a big self-care pat on the back and invite Sister Compassion in to bring you some inner warmth.

Reminding yourself that 'this too shall pass'. It can seem interminably slow to pass and painful but given time, it will.

For those who aren't struggling with that, but may sometimes feel mindfully lazy, it is worth remembering the obvious. When we perform basic hygiene routines, we are getting rid of the old (dirt)which leaves us ready for new experiences. On an energetic level it is a shedding which can leave me feeling lighter.

On the day that I wrote this section, I mindfully went out without a shower or washing my hair; I brushed my teeth. It's rare for me to contemplate this nowadays, but I wanted to eat, that was my prime wellness focus. I felt sticky, like there was an 'oldness' there, as I am so tuned in to my body. When I got back I sat and did some more work, but distractedly conscious of a heaviness of feeling. My mouth felt yucky inside so I brushed my teeth again and had the shower; I immediately felt clearer within myself. Zingy. This is why I do it, and why I so noticeably can't not, and this becomes more ingrained over time as we begin to pay more attention to our physical selves, which then makes us feel better mentally too. I feel like I am prepared for the world, once showered, but if not that I am not fully present or ready.

Sometimes it might be that taking a bath to relax our aching muscles will help, and for those who feel put off by the time it takes to run it, you might set a timer and go off and do other things whilst the bath runs.

## Conscious colour choices

How do your clothes feel on you, Is the texture and fit comfortable for you? What about the colour that you feel drawn to? Can you consciously incorporate colour into your life to help you to balance? See the section on the chakras, in the Energy Hygiene chapter for more information there on those and be aware that colour mostly works in a very subtle way. You may notice the benefits if you are sensitive, and it may be worth working over time with colours that you aren't keen on to help re-balance you.

A brief guide to how colours may help us is red for energy, blood and physical vitality, it is a grounding colour, but contraindicated in cases of inflammation and anger issues. Orange is great for the emotions, energising us and may help to promote a sense of self-worth. Yellow is the colour of happiness, mental stimulation and digestive health. Green can help to balance us as it is on the centre of the spectrum and can help us with grief and chest complaints. Blue is the colour of peace, it has anti-inflammatory properties (think blue plasters) and for helping to centre us in our truth and for throat conditions and thyroid. Turquoise may help with the immune system and can link us to our soul. Purple or indigo is the colour of spirituality, helping us to focus on our third eye, which promotes discernment and non-judgement, and spiritual abilities such as clairvoyance. Lilac and violet can enhance our spiritual connection to the Divine, inspiring and uplifting us and some may find this colour grounding. Black helps us to blend into the background and can absorb energy, whereas white reflects it and contains all the colours of the spectrum, traditionally being seen as a spiritual, cleansing colour. Grey, being a mixture of the two, tends to be a colour of balance, a conservative colour of 'walking the middle path'.

Conscious use of colour for our clothing and working to attain the full spectrum of colour in our lives can help with our self-care. Sometimes this can be quite a transformative feeling, such as putting on a different colour to one that we might normally wear. Other ways that we can use colour and bring more into our lives is via the decor in our home, flowers, the food that we eat and perhaps crystals that we carry, which may all help to rebalance us.

## Meditation / mindfulness

Please see the chapter on this. Focusing on the breath for ten minutes can be a quick recharge, as can taking ten minutes to do nothing. Take time out to check in with your body to see how you feel. What is going on with yourself? How are you? I often do this first thing, and especially on a self-care Sunday and ask myself 'what do I want to do today?' I try to include something that I enjoy and makes my heart sing. I ask my inner exercise guru where I'm going to go for a run today, or if I want to go for a run or a walk or even a complete rest day?

I check in with my inner nutritionist to see what meal my body would like, and often this will come after I have eaten the previous meal because I might not be able to intuitively ascertain what my body would like nice if I plan too much (however, there is also value in planning!). Eating the chosen meal is a mindful process, where even if I do not eat in silence now I pay attention to the flavour, the texture, noticing each mouthful, chewing it and having appreciation for the food that I have and an attitude of gratitude (see counteracting negative thoughts).

# Aromatherapy/ essential oils

Using these in a burner (careful with the candles, or there are electric ones available nowadays), or dissolved in some full fat milk. No more than 5 drops per day in 24 hours and be careful that the oils that you chose suit those that you live with too, both children, adults and pets, especially if they have health conditions or on medication. If you aren't sure ask a qualified aromatherapist or your pharmacist as some essential oils aren't suitable for health conditions such as high blood pressure, diabetes, epilepsy, stroke, etc.

# Holy knickers and new shoes!

Without wishing to pry (remember boundaries!) what is the state of your underwear like? Holes in your knickers, underpants, tights or socks or a faded grey bra with a clasp that doesn't fasten properly? How comfortable are your shoes? Are your clothes a good fit? Self-care, as a day to day drip feed, may be about taking the time to replace the things that need replacing. When we are putting on items of clothing that are old and raggedy, on some level it may feel disheartening and send a message to ourselves that we aren't worthy of new or 'decent' clothing. I appreciate the difficulty in sometimes affording items, but how often do we rack our brains when someone asks us what do we want for a birthday or Christmas, or venture to the sales. For some items, second hand shops also have some great bargains.

# Me time bath

Some of us don't like sitting in dirty water, but others find it a deeply relaxing thing to do. Shutting the door, locking it if you have children, and making it your me time boundary if you can, can be a good recharge. Lighting candles around the bath, reading a book, or listening to some soft relaxing music, especially before bed can also help us to sleep better. The old tradition of Radox in the bath can also be effective for tired muscles, or make up an aromatherapy blend if you know how.

When I was tapering off anti-depressants I used to have a daily bath of patchouli (for grounding anxiety) and bergamot ('winter sun', uplifting antidepressant). Even better, I find adding some magnesium or Epsom salts for aches and pains and calming anxiety work well for me. Rosemary, thyme and lavender help me with aching muscles and if I am in need of real comforting nourishment rose oil, although expensive, is the ultimate oil for self-care; 'because I'm worth it'. Please do be careful and research the essential oils you are using or ask an aromatherapist if you have health conditions. When adding them to the bath dilute them first in 20ml of full fat milk so that they don't sit on top of the water.

## Journaling

This can be a productive release of pent up emotions, to have a good vent if you don't feel able to say things directly or to work out how you might express yourself. Similarly, writing letters of discontent to those that we have issues with can be a form of release. We don't have to send them, but burning them afterwards can just help us to transmute that energy and let it go. Getting it off the chest! I found that writing a letter like this helped me to collect my thoughts. After writing it, the following day the person contacted me. We arranged to go for a walk and I articulated verbally what I'd said in the letter, and was able to let some of that go.

## Eating lunch mindfully

Some of us will work through our lunches in a vague attempt to get home earlier. It doesn't always work that way. Neglecting giving ourselves time to sit and eat, and not having a proper break, can illustrate an inner slave-driver at work, which it would be good to be aware of with regards burn-out! Yes I've been there and done that too. Ask yourself why you aren't giving yourself the time to stop and rest?

## Cup of tea

Just sitting down for ten minutes and having a cup of tea or coffee. Doing nothing else, or putting the TV on for a short while. Having a break from the routine. Or if you do too much sitting maybe getting up and doing some steps! Just sitting quietly and just being for some moments can help to restore and recharge us. Occasionally, if I am running a bit late with appointments, and I have apologised to the client, many have looked at me with an 'it really doesn't matter' expression on their face and conveyed that it was nice to just sit. But we don't often allow ourselves to just do that. Just stop. Setting a timer on your phone can help - and a reminder alarm to remind you to do it!

Or, going out for a cup of tea - let someone else make it for a change, make it an event! For social health, meet a friend and get some of those soul nourishing moments of companionship!

## Laughter

Getting with a friend who you can have a good belly laugh with can work wonders for the soul. Or watching a comedy film, or a comedian or going to a comedy club. I know I often wonder when I do have a good belly laugh, how I can go through phases where it doesn't seem prevalent in my laugh. I'm a lover of cracker jokes, they have to be simple, so I will often share these to a friend's page who has similar humour. There is also laughter yoga, though I've not tried that myself, I can imagine it is quite hilarious! Laughter is a great release and relief of tension!

## Having a lie in

If it appeals, take time to have a lie in on a day when you have the knowledge that you have nowhere to go and nothing to do. You may baulk at that thought because of all your commitments. Can you find a way around it like have someone else to have the children for the night?

## Removing chemicals from your diet and the environment

There is more about this in depth in the nutrition and environment sections. I've felt since a teenager that if I was putting something into my body, that was foreign to it, my body would have to process it and if it was artificial or unnatural, it would be more difficult for the body to do that. Awareness of this started when I was at school and it became apparent that E106 or tartrazine, sunset yellow caused hyperactivity in some children. Over the years, I endeavoured to use products that were as natural as possible. Life isn't black and white, I was a smoker for years too, which didn't help with toxins, but if you are a smoker or a drinker and can't deal with giving that up, I reason that at least taking some pressure off the body by not overloading it may help. Particularly when I had ME I looked at this again, trying to find things that would help me!

Aluminium used to be in many deodorants, I think it still is, and linked with breast cancer, so I stopped using deodorants containing it and rarely use aerosols. I only realised the other day, I often use foil in cooking and have for years, and wondered about the effects of that! So we are always learning and can only do our best and sometimes our bit according to what's right for us. For example, I recently went back to a natural fluoride free toothpaste that also wasn't tested on animals. Unfortunately my tooth sensitivity came back. I stopped using shampoos and face products that contained parabens and SCLS, as well as using natural cleaning products for the house (I could never give up the bleach though, as oxygen bleach didn't work as well and I didn't like the washing powder!) Doing something is better than nothing. As my health improved I have returned to using some products, such as hair-spray, very occasionally.

## Prayer

Many people find the practise of prayer to be a restorative process. I remember one day that I was being particularly hard on myself, because I'd confused appointment times. It doesn't happen very often, but I was feeling my mistake harshly, I couldn't let it go. I asked God to forgive me, as I couldn't forgive myself. Instantly, I felt calm. The power of prayer can be marvellous, the practise of it and how we go about it unique to those of us who chose to do this. I think there are a variety of approaches to this, not that I profess to know that much, so that's all I will say!

## Get honest

Getting honest with yourself may be about facing up and admitting certain truths to yourself. It might be painful, so something we'd rather avoid and perhaps that's OK, you know yourself and sometimes the timing isn't right. However it is, it may serve you to ask yourself whether your job is depleting you because you really don't like it anymore and want to leave. The same may be true of your partner or friend. Or it might be that you do need to face up to certain things within yourself. However, do all with a good dollop of compassion!

## Gratitude

The practise of gratitude can be a great self-care tool. Thinking of the things that we are grateful for in our lives, brings our consciousness to the positives that we do have when sometimes we are feeling worn down and weary. It can promote connectivity and increase our social health when we consider those in our lives that we are grateful to know and be around, accentuating our heart based connections and strengthening our love and appreciation for one another. What we express in gratitude often comes back in a beautiful rebound affect! Listing the ten things that we are grateful for in our life each day, in a journal for example, can be a beautiful, heart opening, uplifting process.

## Switch off your phone or the internet

Having some down time from our all-too-accessible lives and closing the doors on the demands and availability to others can be very calming! When I am doing this I let others know what I'm doing and that I won't be available by phone or email. Sometimes I will go for a few months of Facebook downtime, or a Facebook 'retreat' as I call it.

Sit comfortably with your favourite book, film or music... or... watch your favourite film or series on TV, something that makes you laugh or something that you can have a cry to if you need to release some emotions. Have some real down-time where you can just be and switch your 'doingness' off! Going to the library, or buying a book, or borrowing one. Give yourself time to sit down and delight in the time that you can spend reading. Listening to some music can also be a time well spent upon yourself, listen to your favourite songs or get up and dance and let off some steam and have a good sing!

## Allow yourself to have a nap!

Sometimes this can seem such an indulgence - and something that maybe reserved for Christmas day after lunch! If your body really needs an afternoon nap, surrendering to that feeling every now and then can be a wonderfully nourishing action of self-care. Aaaand relax!

## Cook yourself a delicious meal

Taking time to nourish yourself with good wholesome food that you enjoy, then luxuriating in the time that you have given to yourself to make it and eat it mindfully! Notice how your body feels afterwards.

## Cinema

I would occasionally go to the cinema and think 'I enjoyed that, I should go to the cinema more'. As a SC nudge, I felt inspired to get one of the 'Limitless' cards where you pay a monthly fee and can go to the cinema as often as you like. I mused for several months whether it would be worth me getting, but needing to have a nudge to go out and enjoy myself really was and is a self-care shove! I eventually took up the challenge and do have to push myself at times but I enjoy it when I go, knowing I'm paying for it monthly does give me that extra push.

## Holidays and days out

One of the ultimate forms of SC. To have some purely you, 'down' time and less responsibility is so nourishing. Even just one night away can reset our energy and seem so much longer because we're in a different environment. So more holidays for all of us as part of self-care. When I went to see the rheumatologist and he diagnosed CFS, he gave this as advice: 'have more holidays'. I'd already started to go away by myself in order to explore, develop my adventurous side and build my confidence, as well as recharging myself from work. Particularly by the sea clears my energy. To go away more frequently seemed like a good option when affordable!

However, like myself in the past, we're not always in the position to be able to afford to go away or take time off work. Being self-employed can be particularly difficult in that respect as not only are we bringing in an income during that time, but we are also needing to live and maybe also pay for holiday type experiences during that time. However, the concept of a holiday maybe not about where we go or what we do, it might be about taking that time for ourselves. Having that down time, whether it's at home or going to stay with a friend. Enjoying a walk is free. There are ways of doing things that don't involve finance. And it's always worth asking the Powers that Be, for the finance to be there!

I hadn't been on holiday for so many years due to lack of finance as well as not feeling well or able to do so. However, as I started to feel better, my partner at the time and I had a gas bill refund which paid for my first holiday in years. I cried when I got there! The positive aspect of being self-employed is that finances aren't set to a salary. I now ask that things that I need for my wellbeing are covered - and in the universal flow, they always are. If I need finances for my own treatments, it comes, going away to write, it comes - it can be at the 11th hour (winging it!) but time and time again, I am given what I need. I now trust that process to the point of watching with amusement how the universe is going to provide this time, when it seemingly seems impossible. It is amazing, and inspirational what happens. So try asking!

## Go shopping

Go with the intention of buying yourself something that you might not normally buy, but which demonstrates and sends a message to yourself that you value yourself and care for yourself.

## Paint your nails, have you hair done, visit the barber

Taking time to paint my nails often makes me feel better about myself or go and see a beauty therapist and have a pamper. Taking time to care for ourselves in that way, isn't about vanity (it can be so if we are attached to the way that we look). Taking time to have a pamper can be about appreciating that we are worth it and how that makes us feel. That can be extremely restorative and send a positive message that we value and care for ourselves and that it is ok to do that.

For men, going to a barber for beard trim or a pamper may be worth considering. I think younger males are now more open to self care in this way than previous generations, which is great.

# Hobbies and crafts

Cultivating time for the things that we love to do, that bring us joy and help us to also relax and switch off out of the everyday and ordinary, can be real respite time! Sometimes it can be sociable, such as in a hobby group, like woodcrafting or a sewing group, which adds to our social health too. Knitting and crochet keep hands busy if you find that yours need to be occupied! Counted cross stitch is another popular activity - not to mention card making, decoupage and the list can go on.

As well as maintaining creativity and inviting inspiration into our lives in that way, through the process of 'zoning' out and concentrating on our hobby, we can learn about ourselves during that process. It can be a meditative experience. The recent practise of Mindful colouring and the focus of filling in the mandalas or other pictures in colouring book many people find a relaxing process, time out of the busy world!

## Crosswords, puzzles and sudoku.

I am not very good at maths and with numbers, but I love a game of sudoku, it is a good brain switcher-off for me, perhaps because it engages part of my brain that I don't often use! Solitary switch-offs like solitaire, crosswords and so on can sometimes give us some of that self-care down time we need. Scrabble and other games can also be a sociable events, which forge closer relationships with others (or cause arguments with some! Delete which is applicable for you!).

# Art therapy/ drawing, scribbling and mind doodles

Drawing out our emotions can also be enlightening and help us to see something from another perspective, e.g. what does that smug look on that person's face trigger in me, how could I draw that out and then realising where it comes from in our past for example. Over the years I have produced some pretty fierce pictures of the darkest emotions within me and getting them out did help. It can be quite cathartic.

A little bit of art therapy and drawing how you feel has been mentioned elsewhere in the book and can be a nudge to just get out some of the emotions. You don't have to show others what you have done, in fact from a self-care perspective, doing it just for you, can be even more meaningful.

During lockdown I started running MindDoodle classes on Zoom, a mixture of mindfulness and doodling. Similar to the Zentangle principle, Mindoodles focuses entirely in the moment, rather than an end creation, so we never know what the picture will turn out like. It often surprises people and encourages those to be creative who previously haven't had confidence in their creativity. The focus of creating a doodled picture can bring awareness to our thoughts and self-talk where we can challenge any critical perfectionist ones with kinder compassionate ones.

# Snapshot photography

Macro photography can be wonderfully engaging, taking close ups of objects can really draw us in to the subject and take us out of ourselves and most phones have good cameras on them nowadays, so you don't need expensive photographic equipment to get surprisingly good pictures. It is amazing what we can see when we look close up. I first started this practise years ago inspired by my love of flowers and crystals, it was and is an incredibly relaxing past-time for me. Taking snap shots of items and objects from different angles can also open up how we perceive the world and the things around us. Again, this can give us a little holiday from our minds, taking us out of ourselves and helping us to 'switch off'.

## Oracle & angel cards

Many people find that oracle cards or angel cards can be very encouraging and supportive, so can form a good basis for self-care. They often come with instructions and guidelines how to use them, and as they have increased in popularity, they now come in all manner of forms such as animal, flowers, angels, self-help, equestrian and so forth.

I feel that they are a useful tool to help us to learn to trust our intuition, however it is important to be mindful not to rely on them. During times of confusion they can be supportive or reassuring and help to give us some direction. Used effectively they are best used as a tool to validate or confirm what our intuition is already saying. If we come to rely on them before making decisions or checking in with ourselves, we disempower ourselves and it isn't a healthy way to use them. Rather, use them to help them to tune into the deeper you and your deeper truth.

## Social health

A friend is someone who's loving voice can be heard above the rage of our own destructive self-talk. Social health is our desire and ability to co-exist or be with others; how able we are to integrate into new groups and work within teams in an atmosphere of reciprocity and foster meaningful, caring relationships. It is a willingness and openness to connect, that comes without putting up barriers that keep others out. Understanding how we interact with others, is a large part of self-care. It can open up core issues for us, which when understood and resolved may elicit the struggle that we have in our relationships, so that our relationships are enhanced and strengthened, instead of depleting our energy.

Our relationships with others, as social beings, can function as a survival mechanism. Traditionally, it's often said there is safety in numbers; being outside the group can leave us feeling vulnerable. Being in a group also means that we can share skills in order to move forward in life more efficiently; it is a struggle to do everything 'alone'. 'Fitting in', being accepted and having an adaptability to social situations can also ensure that our needs are met, such as being fed, having a roof over our heads, feeling protected and safe in a group.

## On the outside looking in

I've noticed countless clients, like me, who are on a spiritual path, who say that they have always felt like they are on the outside looking in. They have never felt like they have belonged or been part of 'the group'. I'm a great believer in taking a good look within and asking ourselves honestly, is that because we may have put barriers up ourselves? Maybe we've had to do so to protect ourselves and rather than not feeling like we have fitted in, it can be closer to the truth to say to ourselves, did I really, honestly want to? For me this has been the case, that my judgements of others as an adult, have at times allowed me to stay on the outside of groups and to say that 'I don't feel like I fit in' and 'I don't belong'. This can relieve of us of responsibility whilst we put the blame on others that 'it's their stuff, not mine', or that 'I'm powerless because I don't belong'. Realising, that it's a choice then becomes much more proactive.

## Staying safe

Part of social health is also about our ability to keep ourselves safe from others. It may be a wise intuitive, self-care decision to not socialise with certain groups or certain people, because 'it is their stuff'. In my teens, as a vegetarian, I began making conscious choices to not use products tested on animals. I became a member of BUAV and read information by PETA, etc. On joining a local animal rights group, I could see that the majority of the members were using the group to voice their own anger and issues. It felt unstable and there was a vibe of antagonism which felt dangerous. Despite not wanting to see animals suffer, I also saw that the dairy herd on my boyfriend's farm weren't like the ones that the leaflets were saying were so cruelly treated. This didn't mean to say that some other farms didn't treat their animals cruelly, but there was also a bigger picture. I realised an opinion will often be made strongly with bias to support a cause or point. There can be other sides to the story. I didn't feel like that was my sort of group anyway and in that particular instance leaving the group wasn't about my issues of nervousness, but keeping myself safe.

If we have a family of origin that has been highly dysfunctional and abusive we may have made a decision that 'we never want to be like them' and up the barriers go; so groups can be difficult. We may have many acquaintances, and to all intents and purposes appear to be popular, gregarious people, but actually have very few true friends that we allow to come close to us. Work places can also mirror our family of origin, so we may find that we repeat those experiences that we had in childhood within the organisation that we work for e.g. there may be a culture of covert bullying.

## Social skills

For those who are introverted, highly sensitive people (HSPs), those who have autistic spectrum disorder, who have been in abusive relationships and are challenged with mental health issues such as social anxiety disorder, social health may be well down our list of self-care. It maybe something to fear instead of being seen in a positive light. It was certainly a difficult section for me to write!

We may have poor social skills, without knowing what they are - especially if we have grown up in environments where poor social skills are 'normal'. Our social skills are our ability to interact and communicate with others in both verbal and non-verbal ways, which includes conversing about our mental and emotional experiences. Good social skills involve listening as well as speaking. It's an awareness of social rules, such as 'don't interrupt when another is speaking' as otherwise it can suggest that the person isn't interested in hearing what the other has to say. Good eye contact, being empathetic and staying physically still can indicate that we are interested in another and what they have to say.

On the other end of the spectrum it maybe that we are overly focused on another, to the point of intensity and ask intrusive, inappropriate questions and don't have respect or understanding of their space, bombarding them with texts or phone calls. Having an instinctive intuitive awareness of other people's boundaries - where your space ends and you begin -

is having respect for 'the other' and their differences. A relationship with another is exactly that; *with* another. It isn't 'all about me'. Learning to wait our turn within groups, asking for permission when we do things and being accountable for our actions by recognising when we have made mistakes or are 'out of order', all aid mutuality.

All of these factors can cause us to cut off from others and with such issues, it maybe worth working alongside a counsellor, holistic therapist or a life-coach who may enable you to find tools that will help you to find balance and function and even enjoy being with others - if you so wish to. Sometimes we know deep inside that our poor social health is an imbalance and we would benefit from working through it, whereas at other times or for other people it might be about accepting that it's 'just who we are' or 'its' just how we are for now'.

It's worth considering that we don't always have to change if we struggle with social health. Embracing our uniqueness means that accepting we are who we are and if we are quite happy being in our own company, it's OK. And maybe it's somewhere in between. Like the tides we can go in and out. Years ago, a friend and I joked about how at times we would go through phases where our 'do not disturb' signs would go up. I would not feel an inclination to contact her (and others) and at other times vice versa. We mused that it could be as if our energy does send out our 'invisible cloak' which says 'don't go there', or 'don't think about me', 'I'm hibernating or retreating' or whatever it is we need to do to have some space. Conversely, some of us may find that being by ourselves gives us too much time to ruminate and we need that stimulation or distraction that being with others can provide, as well as the warmth of mutual engagement.

# Find your tribe

As we grow, we inevitably change and because of that our friendships may change. We may come to view the world differently, have different ideas or opinions and find that we no longer resonate with the friends that we are around. This can be quite common when we have a link such as drinking, then a member of that group gives up drinking and wonders how they will now fit in. This is also especially true when people find themselves catapulted onto a spiritual path and begin opening up. We can begin to view the world from a completely different perspective, which can feel alienating, as there are far fewer people around who see the world in this way. However, what tends to happen when we keep being true to ourselves is that people on our path that we have been friends with can fall away. As they do, when one door closes and another opens, we tend to attract new people into our lives who support us on our journey. I do have clients from time to time who have just found themselves in this situation, as I did too, but as we engage in these new activities and ways of being, the Universe does support us. I found particular comfort in the passage called 'A Reason, a season and a lifetime', where it says that some people are with us for a reason in life, others are passing through for a season, then others are our lifetime companions. And it is true.

Many people who are spiritually inclined find there can also be a common theme of difficulties, which then may also trigger a heightened fear of rejection. A turning point for me was when I realised that I didn't like everyone, and that I also had a choice of friendships, and in that way I could wish well the ones I didn't want to be around but also accept that there were also others who might not want to be around me. We have preferences and that isn't always a personal rejection of who we are.

Some of us who are sensitive may need to withdraw from company in order to recharge and recollect ourselves. Elaine Aaron's book, The Highly Sensitive Person is worth a read if you struggle. Being with others can be over stimulating and exhausting, if we are not adept at protecting our boundaries and our energy reserves. Being alone allows us to reset. Those that accept our true nature will accept and support our journey, and us theirs.

True friendship time can be so nourishing. There can be nothing better than sharing our experiences, our joys, our life with someone who mirrors back a warmth and interest in us, as we them. That engagement and love can really turn our lives around sometimes, making a bad day just drain away as we realise what is really important over a vent with a friend. My soul sister Yvonne and I have vent-a-line where we will have a text rant or let off steam moment, just to get stuff off our chest and be heard by another who truly cares.

Going out to the pub or for drinks has been a no go for me over the years. As I've grown, I've learnt to adapt. Rather than try to force a square peg in a round hole, and blame my discomfort about the situations on social anxiety, I've now come to accept I don't feel comfortable or find it enjoyable with too many people in one place, too much noise and when people are being inauthentic, loud and out of control (this used to be as a mask!). It's just not my cup of tea, but I can also appreciate how others enjoy these occasions. Now with the benefit of age, I can say no to things like that, I rarely enjoy them, so why put myself through that? Instead, my social health is to go out with a friend for afternoon tea (which is my cuppa) or a walk or the cinema. As always, it is a tuning in process to see where we are at, how we feel, what works best for us and what is in our best interest. That's true self-care.

## Self-care Sundays

Self-care isn't just for Sundays but it's a good place to start! Self-care Sunday, or whichever allocated day(s) you have off during the week, is about mindfully putting time and effort into paying some attention to yourself. Giving yourself some time, some space or whatever it is that you identify that would charge your battery levels up.

My epiphany about Sunday's being a 'no-planning day' came to me after the realisation that I was in 'doing mode' so much of the week. I'd gone from the illness imposed artificial 'just being' with M.E. to 'always doing'. My logo 'just being' was to remind me of right effort to just be and all the implications of that. Being on the go all the time isn't balanced, even though I was functioning far better than I had in the past, but it was like I'd gone to the other extreme. It was nice to have the energy to do that, but I couldn't sit still, watch TV, nor concentrate and focus on a book. I didn't want to sit and meditate, which is often recommended as helping during times such as this, but the desire and inclination and importantly intuition wasn't there. I believe in listening to that, rather than forcing it. I realised that I needed to re-cultivate or explore the 'being' side of me.

I began to see that I would pack so much in to my life and make many plans to do things and if there was a gap in my diary or spare time *sharp intake of breath* what would I do with it?! It was an anxiety. Although I'd already worked in a good balance of time being 'me' time, such as massage, cinema or walks in nature, my memory was getting worse. My brain felt frazzled. It was difficult juggling and calculating times for my diary at work, it was overwhelming and frying my brains. Fortunately work itself was fine, but the planning wasn't. I figured Sunday was a day that it was practical for me to not do anything, so it became a day to not plan anything or go anywhere even with friends.

Sunday became a day that I would leave open and just tune in to see how I felt and what I wanted to do on that day, and from moment to moment throughout the day. Occasionally it involves events such as a walk or afternoon tea with a friend, but the general rule of thumb is to leave Sundays clear and open, to 'just be'.

It really struck me as I wound down, that this really was what was meant by Sunday as a day of rest; there had always been a self-care plan in place! I began to also appreciate the peace and quiet of Sundays where there is less traffic and busy-ness. I would feel less 'guilty' for not doing or 'achieving' anything. Doing that was an achievement in itself, as you might relate to.

## Give it up!

Being in the human doing habit, it's tempting to say, so what would you do with your self-care Sunday? That, as we've seen, might be encouraging you to plan. But if you can give up planning and see what emerges each Sunday by tuning in to what you want to do, it might be quite surprising how fulfilled you can feel and that not doing can be an achievement in itself!

# Make peace with Christmas

This is an incredibly stressful time of year for many. My therapy room is for that reason a Christmas free zone. Some find the busyness of this time of year, with all the sparkly decorations over-stimulating, coupled with the pressure that many of us put ourselves under and on top of that or at root family of origin issues. I can't advise you how to come to a place of peace with Christmas as we all have different challenges, if we do indeed stress. I can only say that I used to find it an unhappy, anxious time of year but over the year have put boundaries in place, to ensure that it is a day that I engage in activities and with people that I genuinely enjoy being with, rather than feeling like I 'should' be with certain others, because that is what is done.

I have battled with the commercial aspects of Christmas v 'the meaning' (which I'm not entirely sure of either). However, I guess over the years I have reframed Christmas into something that I am at peace with spiritually and what suits me and that tends to be being with people that I love and am grateful to be with and thinking of those that aren't there in that way too. I love cooking so that aspect brings me pleasure too, I don't like being around too many people so keep it quiet and in that way it's relaxed. I particularly enjoy asking for inspiration for gifts that will bring people pleasure, this is fun, as well as asking that the money will be there for those things. I don't tend to buy for the sake of buying, so if I don't feel inspired then I don't push it, but do have fun in the lead up when the inspiration comes through - for me the gifts are a material reflection of my love or caring, or appreciation, for those people.

I spent some years by myself alone at Christmas, because I wanted that space for myself and at times that was tough but something I needed to do. I used to feel that Christmas was a time where the family got together to argue, now I keep it sedate and thoroughly enjoy it. I go for a walk or run in the morning, have a glass of sherry while cooking the meal and my favourite part is the turkey sandwich in the evening and cutting into my home made Christmas cake! Christmas is a time for me where I can feel true gratitude for the people that are in my life - even those that are at a distance, as I can appreciate some better in that way!

# In conclusion

After the journey of looking at the ways that we may be blocking our self-care and why we may do that, we have gone on an expedition into the variety of methods that we can partake in that to nourish our being and restore our soul.

Doing so can also restore our faith in not only ourselves, but in humanity, as well as our spiritual faith. Living a life of depletion is after all no fun! Life is meant to be a joy for us all, it will have its ups and downs and struggles, that is inevitable, but with tools for restoration and repletion now at your fingertips, your recovery from these struggles should be swifter, stronger and, above all, kinder.

Go well! Be well and let your own self-care journey be an inspiration to others to restore their well-being and their soul too. May you walk in beauty.

I'd love to hear how any of the elements in this book have helped you, please email me at selfcare@emmasims.co.uk to tell me about your journey. Reviews of the book will also be much appreciated. Thank you.

# Acknowledgements

To Poppy, bless your little soul.

Thank you to Dawn Knox RSHom for helping me with Poppy, which opened my eyes to homeopathy and the conscious start of my self-care journey.

Susan Winter, Psychic Medium, thanks for sticking your neck out and taking the risk to tell me what you believed to be true and showing me another way. I feel immense gratitude for what you taught me. It turned my perception around, literally.

To my other teachers who inspired me, with passion and care over the years: Dawn Jones, Dawn McGuire, Veronica Schembri, Sylvia Limb. Also, to my shadow teachers, it wasn't an easy journey, but that's taught me much.

I give thanks and gratitude to the therapists and supervisors who have supported my self-care over the years: the team at Gresford Osteopathic Clinic: Paul Baxter, Natasha Franco and Lara Field. Claire Arnold osteopath and supervision. Michelle Welsh BACP for Equine Therapy. Jackie Bates RsHom, Shona Neal MBACP, Dr Jodi Walker. Also, to Jem Harvey, Maxine Johns, Liz Folta & Helen Watkins for massage therapies. And to Penster for teaching me how to hug.

To Helen Watkins, Lauren Garside, Tilly and Scamper for providing the perfect space for the birth of the book.

To Donna McKenzie-Singleton, thanks for asking me what I was laughing at and encouraging my writing. I always hoped this day would come and you'd be reading this.

*To my abundance Queenies in our process of manifesting bright futures. Yvonne Phillips, thank you for being you, your big love, our parallel lives and 'ventaline'.*

*To Kate Strachan, my partner in cake, thanks for 'leading the equine (a!)way', adventures into self-caking, yellow and black tapes on steps, laughter and tears.*

*To Lee Rowlett, thank you for wising me up to questioning other people's intentions and the dandelion wishes (plus our forays into home made self-care face masks).*

*To Susan Masterton, thanks for being in the right place at the right time. You gave me courage and faith to go self-employed and that the path I was walking was not quite as nuts as I was wondering if it might be!*

*To Kate Hutchinson, as you have said transitioning might not always be courageous, rather just something you have to do, but I have enormous respect for you and anyone else who is living a life true to themselves. Thanks for your support during my dark times.*

*To my clients, who by being themselves teach me so much too and inspire me with the courage of their unique journeys.*

### *To my Lockdown Rocks*

*Those who were my rocks and helped to support my self and work-care through the lockdown:*

*Jayne Gabriel my supervisor who provides me with kind, consistent understanding and a gentle grace of strength that you have my back. And you like pink.*

*Jason and Nicola Smalley for their pop up talks, online retreats, inspiration and Facebook refuge in the Way of the Buzzard.*

*To the librarians in my life, Lynda Tunnicliffe, Susan Melancris and Lyn Edwards who have helped to keep my brain going during the times I'd given up on it, by suggesting reads and doing the great job you do, I am so appreciative.*

*To my Mum and to my Dad for shaping me. My mum for the beautiful sunset comments, her love of birds, for 'right speech' and cooking skills (and the family tradition of cake!) and to my Dad for his love of the North Wales countryside, Wordsworth, 'cats, banisters & cheese' and 'Another One Bites the Dust… doo doo doo!'*

*To my sister Andrée for my very first aromatherapy treatment and for the care when I didn't know how to self-care, thank you.*

*Julia Chaplin VA for toiling over the websites, helping me through my technological tantrums, sharing cracker jokes and the suggestion I should write a book. I'll give it another go then!*

*To Judi Selwood of Neighbourhood Economics for deeply listening, business advice and being an anchor. I am truly grateful for our sessions.*

*Stuart Travis, my partner, for your grounding logic and wonderful start to the day hugs. You are my rock.*

*Stu Gallagher at door Eleven designs for my logos and the cover design.*

*Helen Jones for many years of horses, trusting me with the care of Thom and mutual acceptance of silent times in between meeting in shops!*

*To Jan Allan Longshadow, my publisher, for believing in me, thank you.*

# Bibliography

21 day abundance meditation practise, Deepak Chopra

Beyond chocolate, Audrey and Sophie Boss

Breaking down is waking up, Russell Razzaque

Conversations with God, Neale Donald Walsh

Desiderata, Max Ehrman

Dispelling Wetiko, Paul Levy

Eat yourself healthy, Dr Megan Rossi

From out of the darkness, Steve Taylor

Oxford English Dictionary

People of the lie, M Scott Peck

Psychosis or transcendance, Lee Sanella

Spiritual intelligence, Michael Levin

Spiritual unfoldment 1, White Eagle

Tao of Equus, Lynda Kohanov

The highly sensitive person, Elaine Aaron

The slow down diet, Marc Jacobs

Therapeutic hunger, Avnish Bhardwaz & Yvette Maurice

Where you begin and I end, Anne Katherine

Why people don't heal and how they can, Caroline Myss

# Index

# Other Titles by Motiv8.me Press

## Reliving the Past to Release the Present.

### (Traumatic Memories and Letters to my Younger Self)

### Dr. Leo Whyte

Leo seems to be a cheery successful man. He has risen to a senior management level in his career at a young age, has a happy family life and hobbies. What people don't know is the darkness that torments him every day underneath it all.

This is a chronological collection of traumatic memories from Leo's young to middle aged life in north east Scotland. At the end of each section Leo writes a letter to himself at that time with the intent of helping himself look at things differently. He also provides key reflections and lessons learned that are applicable to anyone in similar situations.

# RELIVING THE PAST TO RELEASE THE PRESENT

Traumatic Memories and Letters to My Younger Self

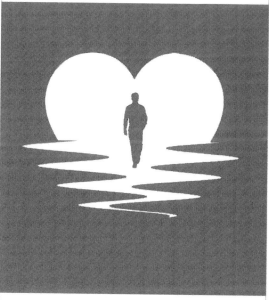

## LEO WHYTE, Ph.D

"A light in the tunnel for those in darkness."

# LIFE SATISFACTION

## A Scientist's Guide to Achieving Health, Happiness and Harmony

### Dr. Leo Whyte

Feeling Stuck? Sick of trying to improve your life only to give up half way or, worse, not feel much better when you get there? Then this approach is for you! In this tale of two halves Dr. Leo presents his no-nonsense Triple 'H' approach to improving your life satisfaction.

In the first part of the book you'll be provided with everything you need to identify the areas to work on for maximum results: you will set goals and install the framework around them for lasting success! In the second part you will read Leo's personal journey using the Triple 'H' approach, documenting the successes and challenges he faced along the way and the astounding results he got in just four weeks.

# LIFE SATISFACTION

## A SCIENTIST'S GUIDE TO ACHIEVING HEALTH, HAPPINESS AND HARMONY

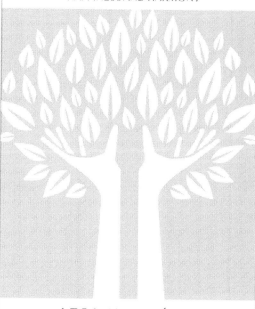

## LEO WHYTE, Ph.D

"An in-depth, accessible and practical approach to getting more out of life."
Motiv8.me Magazine ★★★★★

A Motiv8.me Publication

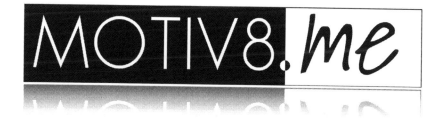

To discover more visit
www.motiv8.me

Printed in Great Britain
by Amazon

53655160R00232